PUBLIC HEALTH IN CHINA SERIES

Series Editor **Liming Li**

Endemic Disease in China

Editor:	Dianjun Sun
Associate Editors:	Shoujun Liu
	Guifan Sun
	Zhizhong Guan
	Xiong Guo

U0294991

People's Medical Publishing House

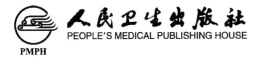

PMPH

Website:http://www.pmph.com/main-en/

Book Title: Endemic Disease in China(Public Health in China Series)
中国公共卫生:地方病防治实践(英文版)

Contact address:No. 19, Pan Jia Yuan Nan Li, Chaoyang District, Beijing 100021, P. R. China, phone/fax: 8610 5978 7584, E-mail: pmph@ pmph. com

First published: 2017
ISBN: 978-7-117-24713-9

Cataloguing in Publication Data:
A catalogue record for this book is available from the
CIP-Database China.

ISBN 978-7-117-24713-9

Printed in The People's Republic of China

Endemic Disease in China

Editor

Dianjun Sun

Director, Center for Endemic Disease Control, Chinese Center for Disease Control and Prevention

Professor,Harbin Medical University

Harbin, China

Associate Editors

Shoujun Liu

Center for Endemic Disease Control, Chinese Center for Disease Control and Prevention

Researcher, Harbin Medical University

Harbin, China

Guifan Sun

Director, Environment and Non-Communicable Diseases Research Center, School of Public Health; Key Laboratory of Arsenic-related Biological Effects and Prevention and Treatment in Liaoning Province

Professor,China Medical University

Shenyang, China

Zhizhong Guan

Director, Key Laboratory of Molecular Biology

Professor,Guizhou Medical University

Guiyang, China

Xiong Guo

Director, Key Laboratory of Trace Elements and Endemic Diseases, National Health and Family Planning Commission of PR of China

Professor,Xi'an Jiaotong University

Xi'an, China

People's Medical Publishing House

Contributors

Dianjun Sun, PhD

Director, Center for Endemic Disease Control,Chinese Center for Disease Control and Prevention

Professor, Harbin Medical University

Harbin, China

Shoujun Liu, PhD

Researcher, Center for Endemic Disease Control, Chinese Center for Disease Control and Prevention

Harbin Medical University

Harbin, China

Ming Li, PhD

Associate Researcher, Center for Endemic Disease Control, Chinese Center for Disease Control and Prevention

Harbin Medical University

Harbin, China

Lijun Fan, PhD

Assistant Researcher, Center for Endemic Disease Control,Chinese Center for Disease Control and Prevention

Harbin Medical University

Harbin, China

Peng Liu, PhD

Associate Researcher, Center for Endemic Disease Control, Chinese Center for Disease Control and Prevention

Harbin Medical University

Harbin, China

Fangang Meng, PhD

Associate Researcher, Center for Endemic Disease Control, Chinese Center for Disease Control and Prevention

Harbin Medical University

Harbin, China

Xiaohui Su, MS

Researcher, Center for Endemic Disease Control, Chinese Center for Disease Control and Prevention

Harbin Medical University

Harbin, China

Zhaojun Zhang, BS

Researcher, Center for Endemic Disease Control, Chinese Center for Disease Control and Prevention

Harbin Medical University

Harbin, China

Zhizhong Guan, PhD

Director, Key Laboratory of Molecular Biology

Professor, Guizhou Medical University

Guiyang, China

Lihua Wang, PhD

Institute for Endemic Fluorosis Control, Center for Endemic Disease Control, Chinese Center for Disease Control and Prevention

Professor, Harbin Medical University

Harbin, China

Xin Li, PhD

Department of Occupational and Environmental Health, School of Public Health; Key Laboratory of Arsenic-related Biological Effects and Prevention and Treatment in Liaoning Province

Professor, China Medical University

Shenyang, China

Yuanyuan Xu, PhD

Professor, China Medical University

Shenyang, China

Bing Li, PhD

Professor, China Medical University

Shenyang, China

Guifan Sun, MS

Director, Environment and Non-communicable Diseases Research Center, School of Public Health; Key Laboratory of Arsenic-related Biological Effects and Prevention and Treatment in Liaoning Province

Professor, China Medical University

Shenyang, China

Guangqian Yu, PhD

Institute for Endemic Fluorosis Control, Center for Endemic Disease Control,Chinese Center for Disease Control and Prevention

Professor, Harbin Medical University

Harbin, China

Lijun Zhao, PhD

Institute for Endemic Fluorosis Control, Center for Endemic Disease Control,Chinese

Center for Disease Control and Prevention

Associate professor, Harbin Medical University

Harbin, China

Xiong Guo, BS

Director, Key Laboratory of Trace Elements and Endemic Diseases, National Health and Family Planning Commission of PR of China

Professor, Xi'an Jiaotong University

Xi'an, China

Feng Zhang, PhD

Associate Professor, Xi'an Jiaotong University

Xi'an, China

Xi Wang, PhD

Assist Professor, Xi'an Jiaotong University

Xi'an, China

Cuiyan Wu, PhD

Assist Professor, Xi'an Jiaotong University

Xi'an, China

Yujie Ning, PhD

Assist Professor, Xi'an Jiaotong University

Xi'an, China

Fangfang Yu, MS

Xi'an Jiaotong University

Xi'an, China

Mohammad Imran Younus, MS

Xi'an Jiaotong University

Xi'an, China

Mikko Juhani Lammi, PhD
Professor, University of Umeå
Umeå, Sweden

Jun Yu, MD
Researcher,Institute of Kashin-Beck Disease, Center for Endemic Disease Control, Chinese Center for Disease Control and Prevention
Harbin, China

Hui Liu, PhD
Associate Researcher, Institute of Kashin-Beck Disease, Center for Endemic Disease Control, Chinese Center for Disease Control and Prevention
Harbin, China

Yanhong Cao, PhD
Researcher,Institute of Kashin-Beck Disease, Center for Endemic Disease Control, Chinese Center for Disease Control and Prevention
Harbin, China

Shuqiu Sun, MD
Professor,Institute of Keshan Disease, Center for Endemic Disease Control, Chinese Center for Disease Control and Prevention
Harbin, China

Hongqi Feng, MD
Associate Professor, Institute of Keshan Disease, Center for Endemic Disease Control, Chinese Center for Disease Control and Prevention
Harbin Medical University
Harbin, China

Jie Hou, PhD

Associate Researcher, Institute of Keshan Disease, Center for Endemic Disease Control, Chinese Center for Disease Control and Prevention

Harbin Medical University

Harbin, China

Acknowledgements

The book is written by nationally renowned experts in the field of endemic disease under the leadership of the Endemic Disease Control Center, Chinese Center for Disease Control and Prevention. The main writers are (in chapters written order) Dianjun Sun, Shoujun Liu, Zhizhong Guan, Guifan Sun, Xiong Guo, etc. Prof. Libin Yang, Prof. Mikko Juhani Lammi, Prof Kewei Wang, Dr. Younas Muhammad Imran and other foreign experts are invited to give English proofreading.

The experts were brainstorming, learning from each other, carefully planning and reviewing, laying out solid foundation for the completion of the book. To achieve the writing style of descriptive language, narrative shows and popular interpretation, the experts and scholars made great contributions to the compilation of the book, they have spent a lot of energy, rearranging the refined materials, designing diagrams, collecting and reshooting clear pictures on the basis of *Endemiology*, a previous Chinese teaching book.

We also have gotten strong support from the Disease Prevention and Control Bureau of National Health and Family Planning Commission, Harbin Medical University, China Medical University, Xi'an Jiaotong University, Guiyang Medical College, and other organizations.

Jun Yan, the chief of the Schistosomiasis and Endemic Diseases Prevention and Control division of Disease Prevention and Control bureau in National Health and Family Planning commission of People's Republic of China, provided valuable

---

Note: Chinese names are conventionally given with the family name preceding the given names. In this book, we retain that convention for national leaders (for example, former Premier Li Peng). Officials, scientists and others are referred to using the Western convention, in which given names precede the family name (for example, Professor Jianbo Yang).

advice. Professor Libin Yang, Kewei Wang in Harbin Medical University, carried out the translation correction of the book. Researcher Zhaojun Zhang, conducted the picture processing, typography and layout.

Hereby I would like to extend my sincerest gratitude to all of you.

Dianjun Sun

Preface

Endemic disease is confined to certain areas and there are dozens in Chinese inland, eight of which have been listed as the national key control endemic diseases. Endemic diseases are serious in China.They are widely distributed, causing severe illness and threatening a large population. Before the founding of People's Republic of China (PRC), endemic diseases were uncontrolled. Few measures were taken to prevent and control them. After the founding of PRC, China attached great importance to the research and control on endemic diseases, classified the prevention and treatment of endemic diseases as the focus of national health work, established the scientific research institutions for the prevention and treatment of endemic diseases, wielded a great deal of human, material and financial resources. After more than 60 years, China has made great achievements on the endemic diseases prevention and control, making the world amazed. During the process, China has accumulated rich experiences on prevention and treatment, summed up complete and effective preventive strategies, which are based on the characteristics of endemic diseases epidemic and prevention work. It is a great treasure that has significant value for the prevention and control of endemic diseases in the past, present and future.

The book focuses on iodine deficiency, endemic fluorosis, endemic arsenic poisoning, Kashin-Beck disease and Keshan disease which are five key national endemic diseases. It has six chapters in total. The first chapter broadly introduces the history of endemic diseases control and prevention in China and the following five chapters systematically and comprehensively introduces the five endemic diseases mentioned above, including the epidemic characteristics, clinical manifestation, diagnosis standards, and the current control situation, preventive strategy, working experience, and successful control cases, etc.

Dianjun Sun

Contents

Acknowledgements ·· xi

Preface ··· xiii

Chapter 1   Introduction ··· 1

    Abstract ··· 1

    1. 1   What is Endemic Disease? ··· 2

    1. 2   How to Classify the Endemic Diseases ··························· 4

    1. 3   Endemic Diseases in China ·· 7

    1. 4   Epidemiological Characteristics of the Endemic Diseases ·············· 14

    1. 5   The History for Endemic Disease Prevention and Control ············ 20

    1. 6   Achievements for the Endemic Disease Control in China ············· 26

    1. 7   The Strategy for Endemic Disease Control and Prevention in
        China ··· 31

    1. 8   The Experience for Endemic Disease Control and Prevention in
        China ··· 36

Chapter 2   Iodine Deficiency Disorders (IDD) ····························· 44

    Abstract ··· 44

    2. 1   The Main Manifestations and Harms of Iodine Deficiency ············ 45

    2. 2   The Story of IDD Discovery ·· 51

    2. 3   Distribution of IDD? ·· 54

    2. 4   Classifications of IDD Endemic Areas in China ················ 58

    2. 5   Prevention Strategies and Measures of IDD? ························ 59

2. 6　IDD Surveillance ·· 65

2. 7　Achievements in IDD Prevention and Control of China ·············· 69

Chapter 3　Endemic Fluorosis ·· 73

Abstract ·· 73

3. 1　General Introduction to Endemic Fluorosis ···················· 73

3. 2　Characteristics of Factors that Influence Endemic Fluorosis ·········· 77

3. 3　What Is Metabolic Pathway and Physiological Role of Fluoride

in Our Body? ·· 84

3. 4　Which Organs or Systems Are Impaired by Endemic Fluorosis? ······ 85

3. 5　Can Endemic Fluorosis Be Diagnosed Clinically? ·················· 92

3. 6　Characterization of the Different Regions of Endemic Fluorosis ······ 95

3. 7　Definition of Regions with Endemic Fluorosis and Different

Degrees of Severity ·· 96

3. 8　Prevention and Control of Endemic Fluorosis ···················· 97

3. 9　Can Endemic Fluorosis Be Treated? ···························· 106

3. 10　History of Control of Endemic Fluorosis in China ················ 107

3. 11　The Achievements of China's Programs for Prevention and

Control of Endemic Fluorosis ································ 111

Chapter 4　Endemic Arsenic Poisoning ·································· 117

Abstract ·· 117

4. 1　Background of Endemic Arsenic Poisoning in China ·············· 118

4. 2　The Classification and Geological Environment of Endemic

Arsenicosis Areas ·· 121

4. 3　Epidemiology of Endemic Arsenic Poisoning in China ·············· 125

4. 4　Mechanism of arsenicosis ································ 130

4. 5　Clinical Manifestations ································ 130

4. 6　Diagnostic Criteria of Endemic Arsenicosis in China ·············· 135

4. 7　Definition and Classification of Endemic Arsenicosis Area ········ 138

4. 8　China's Approach for Prevention and Control of endemic

arsenicosis ·· 139

4.9 China's Achievement and Experience ······························ 146

Chapter 5 Kashin-Beck Disease (KBD) ···························· 150

Abstract ·· 150

5.1 The Discovery of The Disease ······························· 150

5.2 Epidemiology and Disease Characteristics ··················· 158

5.3 Etiology and Epidemic Mechanism ······················· 160

5.4 Clinical Manifestation and Diagnosis ······················· 173

5.5 Prevention and Control of KBD ·························· 181

5.6 The Treatment and Its Unified Evaluation Standard for KBD ······ 186

5.7 More Experience of Prevention and Control of KBD ··············· 198

Chapter 6 Keshan Disease ································· 212

Abstract ·· 212

6.1 The Discovery of KD ································· 213

6.2 Epidemiology ····································· 214

6.3 Etiology ······································· 218

6.4 Clinical Manifestation and Diagnosis ······················· 220

6.5 Cardiac Histopathology ······························ 232

6.6 Therapies ······································· 240

6.7 Prevention Measures ································· 245

6.8 Surveillance ····································· 249

6.9 Achievements ····································· 253

6.10 Valuable Experiences in Control and Prevention of KD ············ 259

Chapter 1

Introduction

Dianjun Sun

Abstract

Endemic disease is a generic term for the diseases with endemic or regional features, which is closely related to natural environment, human life and production. China is severely affected by endemic diseases. Multiple endemic diseases exist in China, of which some are unique but others also exist in other countries. The endemic diseases are prevalent in all provinces of China and threaten nearly 100 million residents. Since the foundation of P. R. China, the government has attached great importance to the control and prevention of endemic diseases. The leadership and research institutions have been established nationwide. Huge amounts of funds have been invested. Many experts have been organized for cross-disciplinary research and the research results have been used to guide the control and prevention of endemic diseases. Especially in recent years, the Chinese government set up special projects and invested over 100 billion RMB to implement appropriate prevention and control measures in the endemic diseases areas. Through continuous efforts in the control and prevention over 60 years, the endemic diseases in China have been effectively controlled, and rich experiences have been obtained. This chapter describes the definition, classification and epidemic characteristics of endemic diseases, as well as the history, achievements, strategies and experiences in the control and prevention of endemic diseases in China.

China was once one of the worst-affected countries by endemic diseases in the world, characterized by multi-types, high prevalence, serious public health hazard and wide distribution. There were not only geochemical endemic diseases and natural focus endemic diseases but also Chinese unique endemic diseases. The number of affected population ranked first in the world, with ten million people suffering endemic diseases and one or more types of endemic diseases distributed in every province of China. The occurrence and prevalence of endemic diseases brought serious detriment to the health, life and production of the residents living in endemic disease areas, and affected national prosperity and local economic development. Since the foundation of P.R. China in 1949, Chinese government had deeply concerned about and attached great importance to the prevention and control of endemic diseases, established the leader group and professional institutions, deployed tremendous human resources and material resources, and carried out scientific research and prevention and control of endemic disease. This is an outstanding feature of Chinese endemic disease control, which is different from other countries in the world. All measures contributed to the containment of epidemics and hazard of endemic diseases in China, and abundant experience had been accumulated ever since. To date, the overall trend of endemic diseases in China has been controlled and some types of endemic diseases have even approached a level of total eradication. Endemic diseases also occur in other countries and are mainly distributed in the underdeveloped countries and regions where there are no centralized administrative organizations for its prevention and control. Currently, Chinese prevention and control for endemic disease is top-ranked worldwide. However, the natural environment for endemic disease prevalence is difficult to be changed, and it is one of major public health issues in the vast countryside of China. Especially, endemic diseases are relatively severe in some regions of western China. Therefore, endemic diseases are still a crucial issue threatening Chinese health.

1.1 What is Endemic Disease?

There are several kinds of described concepts about endemic diseases. Professor John M. Last, a renowned Canadian epidemiologist who was commissioned by the International Epidemiological Association to compile an epidemiological dictionary, defined endemic disease as the constant presence of a disease or infectious agent within a given geographic area or population group, and it might also refer to the usual prevalence of a given disease within such area or group. Professor Jianbo Yang, a well-known Chinese expert in Epidemiology/Endemiology, considered endemic disease as one confined to certain regions. Professor Shangpu He, a Chinese epidemiologist, described it as one which frequently reoccurred in some regions without inputting new cases from outside. In the endemic volume of China's first set of Medical Encyclopedia, it defined endemic disease as one which was relatively stable and frequently reoccurred within certain regions. These concepts all emphasize that the diseases' occurrence is region-restricted or endemic.

The concepts mentioned above changed the incomplete and narrow understanding that endemic disease was an adaptive disease (tellrisum) closely related to local environment, i.e., the pathogeny existed in the water and soil of endemic areas. Certain elements or its compounds in the water and soil of endemic areas are excessive or insufficient, and they act on human body through food and water intake. Along with in-depth study, it has become more and more limited only to regard endemic disease as tellrisum. For example, lifestyle-related and natural focal endemic diseases could not been classified into the endemic category. Therefore, the diseases with endemic characteristics caused by various reasons should belong to the category of endemic disease, according to the research and the current situation of endemic prevention and control in China.

At present, a suitable definition for Chinese endemic disease is that all the diseases characterized by endemic occurrence should belong to the category of endemic disease.

From clinical perspective, endemic diseases do not appear as an independent disciplinary system. For example, Keshan disease is a cardiovascular disease and Kashin-Beck disease is an osteoarthritis disease. This classification is only from the therapeutic point of view and does not seize the essence of endemic diseases. The most prominent feature of endemic disease is the endemic occurrence, while the endemicity depends on the local complicated natural and social environment. In this sense, the endemic disease is a very typical environment-related disease, which is preventable but cannot be cured. And the core is that the pathogeny should be found in the endemic environment (disease-causing substances). Comprehensive environment-reform measures should be taken to block the entrance of pathogenic substances into the body. Government leadership and multi-department cooperation should be reflected in the prevention and control. Consequently, endemic disease should belong to the category of preventive medicine with its own unique research contents and purposes.

1.2 How to Classify the Endemic Diseases

Endemic diseases can be classified into four categories according to the pathopoiesis, including geochemical diseases, natural focus diseases, specific lifestyle-related diseases and endemic diseases of unknown causes, as shown in Table 1. Once the causes become clear, the endemic diseases of unknown causes will be listed into the other three categories. In addition, there is also endemic genetic disease in China, such as β- thalassemia, but it has never been incorporated into the management for endemic disease prevention and control.

1.2.1 Geochemical Disease

What is geochemical disease? Some chemical elements from the surface of the earth crust are unequally distributed during the natural formation of the Earth, coupled with human life and production activities, and combined into different categories of certain chemical compounds of water, soil, plants, air and coal which are closely related to human survival. Some elements in an appropriate amount are necessary to human health. Once the population is exposed to the environment with excessive or insufficient intake of these chemical elements for a long term, the health is affected and relative diseases may occur. Therefore, geochemical diseases are outcomes due to the effect and impact originating from geochemistry. Geochemical diseases mainly include iodine deficiency disorders, drinking water type fluorosis, drinking water type arsenicosis, endemic selenium poisoning and endemic acute barium poisoning (Bi disease), etc. Owing to the evidently regional distribution, these diseases are classified into endemic diseases in China.

1.2.2 Natural Focus Disease

What is natural focus disease? In the 1930s, Pavlovsky, an academician of the Academy of Sciences in the former Soviet Union, proposed a theory of natural focus disease. To understand natural focus disease, we need to know what natural foci are. The natural foci refer to the areas where a certain pathogenic agent is preserved in wild animals on a long-term basis and causes the disease prevalence among the animals. The natural foci consist of pathogenic agent, susceptible animals and spread vectors. Under certain conditions, human being may be infected after entering the natural foci, and the disease spreads from wild animals to human, hence called natural focus disease. Because there is a specific ecological environment in natural foci, this determines the endemism of natural focus disease, including schistosomiasis, plague, brucellosis, tick-borne encephalitis, malaria, filariasis, hydatid disease, etc.

1.2.3 Particular Production and Life Style-related Disease

Just as its name implies, particular production and life style-related disease is caused by certain human production or living habits. For example, coal-burning fluoride poisoning and coal-burning arsenic poisoning are due to long-term burning of high-fluoride or high-arsenic coal bin in indoor stoves without sufficient ventilation, and excessive fluoride or arsenic contaminates the indoor air and food; brick-tea type fluorosis is due to long-term consumption of brick tea with high-fluoride content and accumulation of excessive fluoride in the body; and botulism is a kind of poisoning caused by customarily eating homemade soy products, etc.

Among the diseases listed in Table 1, there are four unique endemic diseases in China, including coal-burning type fluorosis, coal-burning type arsenicosis, brick-tea type fluorosis and Pazhi disease (a kind of endemic osteoarthritis occurring only in Sichuan province, China). Keshan disease (KD) and Kashin-Beck disease (KBD) are mainly distributed in the territorial boundary areas of the Northeast China, in which two endemic diseases occurred in history. In Siberian region bordered by Russia and the Northeast China, there was the prevalence of Kashin-Beck disease, which was controlled by the implementation of changing grain source early in the 1960s. In some northern areas of North Korea bordering the northeast China, there was the prevalence of Kashin-Beck disease and Keshan Disease, but no new report has been published. Iodine deficiency disorders, endemic fluorosis and arsenicosis all belong to geochemical endemic diseases that occur in many countries worldwide, and the situation is even worse in some underdeveloped countries. Iodine deficiency disorders are mainly distributed in the developing countries, particularly some underdeveloped and poor countries in Africa, Asia and South America. The well-known epidemic areas of iodine deficiency disorders include Asian Himalayas, European Alps and Pyrenees, the basin of Five Great Lakes in North America, the Andes in South America, the African Congo Basin and Papua New Guinea in Oceania. Endemic fluorosis prevails in more than 50 countries and regions worldwide, such as India, Bangladesh, China, Thailand and Sri Lanka in Asia, Russia, Bulgaria and Italy in Europe, Morocco, Algeria, Kenya and Tanzania in Africa, the United States of America, Canada and Argentina in America, Australia in Oceania, etc. Endemic fluorosis in these countries is caused by drinking high-fluoride containing water. Over 50 million people worldwide are estimated to be exposed to arsenic with a concentration above 0.05mg/L in drinking water, and the world's worst regions of endemic arsenicosis are distributed in Bangladesh, Indian West Bengal and China. The affected population is up to 30 million in Bangladesh alone.

Table 1.1 Classification of Endemic Diseases and Main Types

Classification	Main types
Geochemical endemic diseases	Iodine deficiency disorders (IDD), Drinking-water type fluorosis, Drinking-water type arsenicosis, Endemic selenium poisoning, Endemic acute barium poisoning (Bi disease), etc.
Natural focus endemic diseases	Schistosomiasis, Plague, Brucellosis, Tick-borne encephalitis, Malaria, Filariasis and Hydatid disease, etc.
Particular production and life style-related endemic diseases	Coal-burning type fluorosis, Brick-tea type fluorosis, Coal-burning type arsenicosis, Kuru disease (caused by eating the brain of the dead), Burning sensation disease (gossypol poisoning caused by eating cottonseed oil), Botulism (mainly by eating homemade soybean products and other fermented food), etc.
Endemic diseases of unknown etiology	Keshan disease (KD), Kashin-Beck disease (KBD), Pazhi disease, Black foot disease, etc.

1.3 Endemic Diseases in China

Endemic diseases are seriously prevalent in China, and the residents out of 31 provinces are suffering their harm at different degrees (Fig. 1.1). Eight kinds of diseases were once included in the main endemic disease management for prevention and control, including Schistosomiasis, Keshan disease, Kashin-beck disease, iodine deficiency disorders, endemic fluorosis, endemic arsenicosis, plague and burcellosis. With the change of administration function, Schistosomiasis, Plague and Burcellosis were put under the category of communicable diseases. Now, only the rest five diseases are still under the endemic disease management for prevention and control.

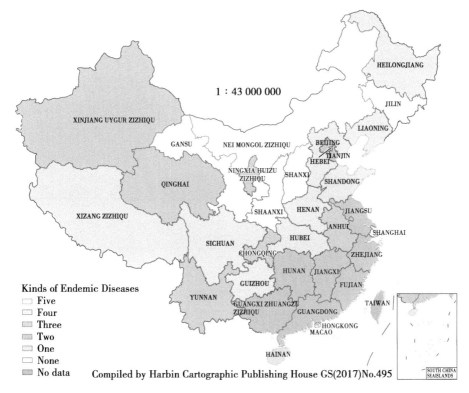

Fig. 1.1   Distribution of endemic diseases in China

1.3.1   Iodine Deficiency Disorders (IDD)

IDD is a syndrome induced by insufficient iodine intake due to the iodine deficiency of external environment. Decreased secretion of thyroid hormone is the main pathogenesis. Its main damage to population health is manifested by different degrees of brain development retardation, which affects the quality of life of national population and is a significant public health problem. The IDD has a wide disease-spectrum, including endemic goiter which is the most common one, endemic cretinism, subclinical cretinism, neonatal congenital hypothyroidism, congenital anomalies, deaf-mutism, premature birth, miscarriage, stillbirth, etc.

The IDD is the most widely distributed and the most prevalent disease in the world. Iodine is an active non-metallic element, existing in compound form in nature and is rare. The content of iodine in the crust of earth is ranked at the forty-seventh. The global iodine deficiency environment is related to the forth glacial epoch which began about two million to three million years ago, and ended in 10,000 to 20,000 years ago. Although the forth glacial epoch lasted very long, the replacement of cold weather and warm weather still existed, and the glacier dissolved repeatedly. Because of the flood scouring, especially the inundation at the end of glacial epoch, the iodine-rich mature soil was washed away and the iodine in the new soil formed from rock was less than 1/10, which led to the iodine deficiency worldwide. In general, the closer ocean the soil is, the higher content of iodine it is. The farer away ocean the soil is, the lower iodine content it is (Table 1.2). However, some studies show that the impact of the marine environment on iodine content of the soil might not extend far inland. In China, iodine deficiency covers large areas of its natural environment. (Fig. 1.2). The iodine content is lower not only in the soil but also in drinking water. Except for Shanghai, IDD is prevalent in 30 provinces and regions. In 1990s, due to iodine deficiency there were about eight million patients with endemic goiter and 187 thousand patients with endemic cretinism in China. Although the natural environment in most areas of China is short of iodine, China has the largest high iodine areas in the world, which are distributed in 115 counties of nine provinces and about 30 million residents are threatened.

1.3.2　Endemic Fluorosis

Endemic fluorosis is a geochemical disease in specific geographical environment. It is a cumulative chronic toxicity in the whole body due to a long-term exposure to excessive quantity of fluorine in drinking water, air and food. Dental fluorosis and

Table 1. 2   The iodine content in the soil of coastal and inland areas(mg/kg)

Sample source	Range of iodine content	Mean	Reference
Coastal areas			
Northwestern Norway	5.4-16.6	9	Lag and Steinnes (1976)
Wales	1.5-149	14.7	Fuge (1996)
Ireland	4.2-54	14.7	Fuge (unpublished data)
Inland areas			
Eastern Norway	2.8-7.6	4.4	Lag and Steinnes (1976)
Wales/England	1.8-10.5	4.2	Fuge (1996)
Missouri of USA	0.12-5.6	1.3	Fuge (1996)
USA[a]	<0.5-9.6	1.2	Shacklette and Boerngen (1984)

[a] Including some samples of coastal areas

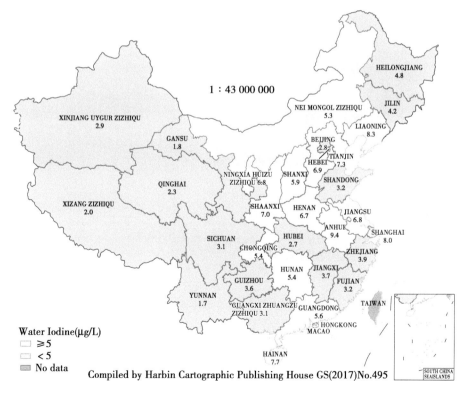

Fig. 1. 2   Distribution of iodine content in drinking water of China.

skeletal fluorosis are the essential clinical manifestations of endemic fluorosis. Fluorine was found about 200 years ago, which has the strongest electronegativity and strong oxidation ability. The fluorine is chemically very active, can replace other halogens from compounds, combines with lots of metal elements under normal temperature, and almost reacts with all elements under high temperature. Thus, it exists in the form of compound instead of element in nature. At the same time, the vast majority of inorganic fluoride can be dissolved in water and has high melting point and boiling point. So, the migration ability of fluorine is very strong, making it widely exist in rock, soil, water, air and animals, and easily be obtained by human. In order to prevent the prevalence of fluorosis, 1.5mg/L, the upper limit value of fluoride content recommended by WHO in drinking water is adopted in many countries. The national standard of China and India is 1.0mg/L, and it is relaxed to 1.2mg/L in China for the small size central water supplies ($<1000m^3$ provided per day) in the countryside (Table. 1.3).

Table 1.3   Provisions and Recommended Values for the Fluoride in the Drinking Water by Some International Organizations and Counties

Organization or country	Standard category	Concentration (mg/L)	Note
World Health Organization	Recommendation	1.5	Recommended in 2004
Environmental Protection Agency of USA	Primary standard	4.0	Compulsory
Environmental Protection Agency of USA	Secondary standard	2.0	Optional, to prevent dental fluorosis
European Union	Maximum allowable concentration	1.5	Provision of 1998
Canada	National standard	1.5	
India	National standard	1.0	From 1.5 to 1.0 in 1998
China	National standard	1.0	
Tanzania	National standard	8.0	Temporary standard

Chinese drinking water type fluorosis is distributed in 1,137 counties of 28 provinces, threatening about 87.28 million residents. The coal-burning type endemic fluorosis is distributed in 173 counties of 13 provinces, threatening about 33.76 million residents. The brick-tea type fluorosis is distributed in 304 counties of 7 provinces, threatening about 16 million residents.

1.3.3 Endemic Arsenicosis

Endemic arsenicosis is a chronic systemic poison induced by excessive arsenic intake due to overtime exposure to high level arsenic in the environment. Its main pathogenesis is skin depigmentation or hyper-pigmentation, palmoplantar keratoderma and canceration. Arsenic (As) is a primary element which exists in the environment and mostly in the form of compounds, such as hydride, oxide, sulfide of arsenic and so on. According to the source of arsenic, humans are exposed through four pathways: life contact, occupational exposure, environmental pollution, and iatrogenic intake. Among them, life contact is the primary way to induce the occurrence of endemic arsenicosis. In life contact, endemic arsenicosis is mainly induced by drinking arsenic-rich groundwater, which is basically the same condition in all the arsenic-poisoning countries in the world. Moreover, besides the drinking water type arsenicosis, there is another type of endemic arsenicosis in the affected remote mountainous areas in China. Since local residents burn high arsenic coal, polluting the air and food in the room and inducing chronic arsenic poisoning, it is called coal-burning type arsenicosis (Fig. 1.3). This type of arsenicosis is unique in China, only found in Guizhou and Shanxi provinces, affecting 1.22 million residents from 12 counties. The drinking water type arsenic poisoning areas where patients are found cover 885 villages of 62 counties in 10 provinces, affecting about 632 thousand residents. Although the arsenic-rich drinking water is found in 2015 villages of 142 counties from 14 provinces, affecting about 1.43 million residents, no patient has been diagnosed with arsenicosis.

1.3.4 Kashin-Beck Disease (KBD)

KBD as an endemic disease is characterized by multiple chronic osteoarthropathy whose pathological changes are degeneration, necrosis and secondary osteoarthritis in

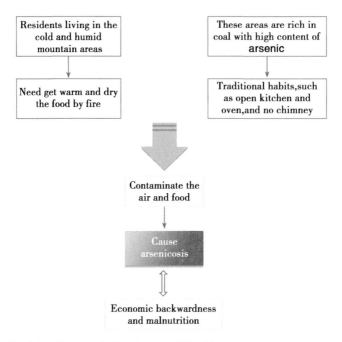

Fig. 1.3　The onset sketch map of Coal-burning type arsenicosis.

children's articular cartilage of the extremities (Fig. 1.4). The serious patients are manifested by short height, deformity and disability for their life. At present, the etiology and pathology of KBD remain under investigation. The KBD is distributed from Sichuan-Tibet region to the northeast of China, and spreads to the eastern Siberia of Russia and the northern mountainous area of North Korea. No KBD patients occur in other regions of the world. In China, the KBD is diagnosed among 21,436 villages of 378 counties in 13 provinces, affecting about 21.97 million residents.

1.3.5　Keshan Disease (KD)

KD is an endemic myocardial disease (Fig. 1.5). In 1935, it attracted the world's attention for the first time due to its big prevalence in Keshan County of Heilongjiang Province of China, hence named Keshan Disease. The main pathological characteristics of KD are myocardial parenchymal degeneration, necrosis and scar formation, myogenic dilatation, heart enlargement, and thinner wall. The chief clinical manifestations are cardiac arrhythmia and cardiac decompensation, which is further classified into acute, sub-acute, chronic and latent types. The KD is an independent,

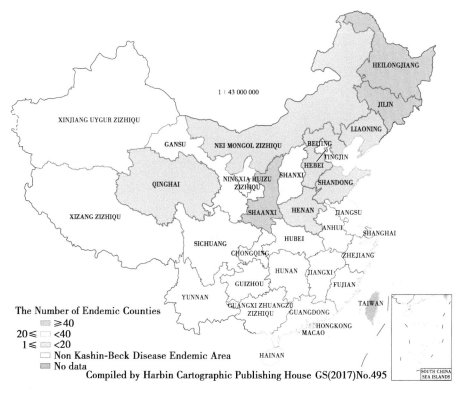

1 : 43 000 000

The Number of Endemic Counties
≥40
20≤ <40
1≤ <20
Non Kashin-Beck Disease Endemic Area
No data

Compiled by Harbin Cartographic Publishing House GS(2017)No.495

Fig. 1.4　The distribution of Kashin-Beck disease in China.

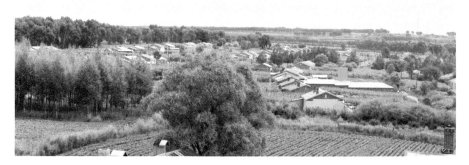

Fig. 1.5　The place where KD was first found—the natural landscape of Keshan county, Heilongjiang province.

primary myocardial disease. It is distributed in 327 counties from 16 provinces in China, affecting about 59. 53 million inhabitants.

1.4 Epidemiological Characteristics of the Endemic Diseases

1.4.1 Distribution of Endemic Areas

The most prominent character of epidemic diseases is that they happen in the relatively steady location. This is because the development of every endemic disease is closely related to its own pathogenic factor which is distributed parochially in restrictive area. Living in the endemic disease area is one essential condition in diagnosis standards of most endemic diseases. The endemic diseases are often distributed in such areas, looking like a "focus", "patchy" or "strip" shapes,

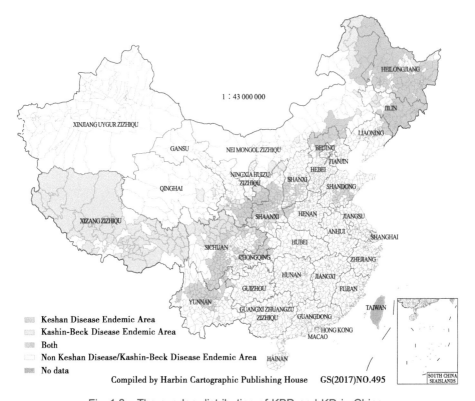

Fig. 1.6　The overlap distribution of KBD and KD in China.

including KD, KBD, endemic fluorosis, endemic arsenicosis, and so on. Among them, KD and KBD overlap in some areas (Fig. 1.6). Mild endemic disease area and non endemic disease area may coexist in the same patchy region. Taking endemic arsenic poisoning as an example, the arsenic levels of well water have significant differences in the same village. The high arsenic wells and the normal arsenic wells as neighbors may just be separated by a wall. So, endemic arsenic poisoning is distributed in such areas of small focus or punctate shape (Fig. 1.7).

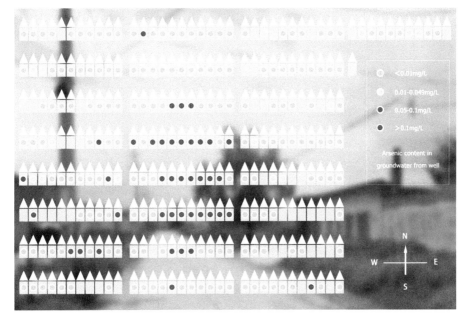

Fig. 1.7   The distribution of wells with different arsenic concentrations in the same endemic village

The onset and prevalence of endemic diseases are closely related to geographical environment. KD and KBD are distributed in the middle or low altitude mountain areas, hilly land and part of its adjacent plain area with continental climate, which is relatively wet and there is a large temperature difference between night and day. The more serious IDD occurs in the regions with sloping terrain, in which there are more rain causing soil erosion. The prevalence of IDD in mountainous areas is more serious than in hilly areas, so are in hills than in plains and in inland than in coastal areas. The drinking water type fluorosis is distributed in the low-lying areas with worse groundwater runoff conditions or high fluorine rocky areas. The drinking water type arsenicosis is distributed in the basin close to mountains, lower terrain of piedmont alluvial and alluvial plain, or mining areas rich in arsenic (Fig. 1.8).

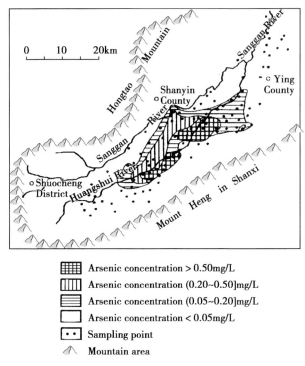

Arsenic concentration > 0.50mg/L
Arsenic concentration (0.20~0.50]mg/L
Arsenic concentration (0.05~0.20]mg/L
Arsenic concentration < 0.05mg/L
Sampling point
Mountain area

Fig. 1.8 Map showing the distribution of arsenic-bearing groundwater in Datong Basin

1.4.2 Population Prevalence

Agricultural residents in rural areas are the high-risk population of endemic diseases, especially KSD and KBD. The major patients are self-sufficient agricultural population, and the non-agricultural population is rarely affected in the same area. As to other kinds of endemic diseases, the rural population is also easily to contact pathogenic factors without exception, such as schistosomiasis, plague, brucellosis, IDD, endemic fluorosis and endemic arsenicosis. Why do endemic diseases not prevail seriously in cities? Firstly, the economy and culture are developed in urban life and the sanitary condition in city is better than that in other areas, while it is almost impossible for the natural focal disease foci. Secondly, the quality of urban drinking water must be satisfied with the national health standards, in which fluoride and arsenic do not exceed the national standard. Thirdly, the living levels of urban residents are higher, and they can intake trace elements and other nutrients through a variety of ways. Therefore, the residents living in the city are rarely exposed to the pathogenic factor of endemic diseases.

The onset age of endemic diseases is different. The mainly susceptible groups are women with childbearing age and children with age between preschool and ablactation(Table 1.4). Children and teenagers are susceptible to KBD, while adults rarely suffer from KBD. High-risk groups of IDD are babies of 0-2 years old, children, pregnant women and lactating women. Endemic fluorosis and endemic arsenicosis are cumulative diseases of poisons. It is common that the older the patient is, the more serious the illness is. But dental fluorosis develops only in initiation period of dental caries, it doesn't reoccur in children who have grown permanent teeth after they migrate into endemic areas. Of other endemic diseases, the age of the vulnerable population depends on when and how often they are exposed to pathogenic factors.

Table 1.4   The Gender Contrast of Acute KD in Heilongjiang Province from 1955 to 1966

Year	55	56	57	58	59	60	61	62	63	64	65	66
Male	23.4	26.6	25.1	26.0	27.9	36.6	37.3	34.6	29.9	30.2	30.1	34.5
Famle	76.6	74.4	74.9	74.0	72.1	63.4	62.7	65.4	70.1	69.8	69.9	65.5
summation	100.0	101.0	100.0	100.0	100.0	100.0	100.0	100.0	100.0	100.0	100.0	100.0

There are no significant gender differences in endemic diseases, except for KD, IDD and skeletal fluorosis, which are related to gender, presenting a phenomenon of more women cases than men patients suffering the illness. Female patients also have a more serious state of the illness. In ethnically mixed areas, differences of endemic disease incidence are not significant among different ethnic groups if their production and life styles are similar.

Endemic diseases are often prevalent in poor areas, too. The poorer areas are, the more serious the disease is. Statistics in 1996 showed that 576 counties out of 592 national-level poverty counties were identified as severe areas of endemic disease, accounting for 97.3% of total disease areas.

Clustering phenomenon occurs within family for some endemic diseases, that is, there are more than two patients one after another in same family(Fig. 1.9). Residents living in the northern endemic disease areas call it "snap diseases". Most of the families are at low income levels. Some immigrated settlers from other places have poor living conditions and many children. The clustering phenomenon of disease in a family is obviously existed in KD, KBD and endemic arsenicosis. Some endemic diseases have the phenomenon of bullying foreign immigrants, of whom prevalence of the disease (i.e., KD, KBD and endemic fluorosis) is clearly higher than that of local residents under the same production and living conditions after their migration from non-endemic disease areas into the endemic disease areas.

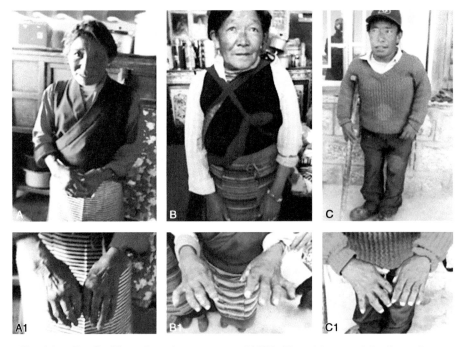

Fig. 1.9　Family Clustering phenomenon of KBD (the sisters and brother of one family in Nimu county, Lasa, Tibet, 2011). A: elder sister (Degree Ⅱ KBD patient). B: younger sister (Degree Ⅲ KBD patient). C: younger brother (Degree Ⅲ KBD patient). A1: The hand of Elder sister. B1: The hand of younger sister. C1: The hand of younger brother.

1.4.3　Seasonal variation

Seasonal variation is one feature of endemic diseases since its pathogenic factor distribution and specific popular mechanism vary in different seasons. Namely, it is easy for people to expose to pathogenic factors or they are attacked or infected a while ago, and they eventually get the disease in one season after an incubation period and development process of the disease. Taking KD as an example, in the northern disease areas, the common season of acute KD is cold winter, from November to next April (Table. 1.5), while as to subacute KD it is in hot summer, from July to August. Prevalent seasons of KBD are winter and spring. The onset of geochemical endemic disease is not obviously related to season but to climate. Schistosomiasis can be infected in the whole year, of which the chances of infection are higher in spring and summer, but lower in winter. The epidemic season of human plague mainly depends on the seasonal variation of rodent plague in all kinds of foci. Epidemic peak of hibernating rodent squirrel and marmot plague is from July to September, while long claw sand plague is in all four seasons, of which the first peak is from April to May and the second peak is from October to November. Brucellosis can occur in any month throughout the whole year, but it is more frequent in spring and summer.

Table 1.5　The Monthly Constituent Ratio of Acute KD from 1963 to 1974 in Fanrong Township, Fuyu County, Heilongjiang province

Onset month	1	2	3	4	5	6	7	8	9	10	11	12
Incident number	144	66	57	40	9	2	1	2	1	2	22	62
Constituent ratio %	35.2	16.2	13.9	9.8	2.2	0.5	0.3	0.5	0.3	0.5	5.4	15.2

Some endemic diseases also have the phenomenon of prevailing year, due to changes in natural environment and production and living conditions. If the conditions which cause the occurrence of endemic diseases are completely removed, the diseases can be controlled to a lower level or even completely eliminated. Like schistosomiasis, its prevalence is greatly affected by rainfall and flood. During 1990s, floods spread in Yangtze River Basin, causing a rise of the water for a long time and large flooded areas, increasing areas of oncomelania breeding and expanding disease areas. So, it may be easier for schistosomiasis to prevail in the year of more rainfall or some years following a flooding.

1.5 The History for Endemic Disease Prevention and Control

More than two thousand years ago, in *Inner Canon of the Huangdi-SuWen* mentioned the relationships between diseases and water, soil and climate conditions. Schistosomiasis once raged in China about two thousand years ago. During 1970s, schistosome eggs were found in the livers and intestinal walls of ancient corpses from Western Han Dynasty, which were unearthed in Changsha of Hunan Province and Jingzhou in Hubei Province. As early as the Sui Dynasty, "lymphadenectasis", which was bubonic plague, was already documented in *General Treatise on the Cause and Symptoms of Diseases* by Doctor Yuanfang Chao, and in *Thousand Pieces of Gold Formulae* by Doctor Simiao Sun during the same period. *Classic of Mountains and Rivers* in the seventh century BC proposed that goiter was a kind of endemic disease, and Doctor Hong Ge in the third century AD in Jin Dynasty used seaweed and kelp to treat this disease. Fluorosis was documented in *Regimen Theory* by Doctor Kang Ji in Jin Dynasty, who wrote down "Teeth of inhabitants were yellow who lived in Shanxi Province". He noticed the geographical role in the occurrence of dental fluorosis. KBD and KD were identified later. KBD was written in *The Annals of Anze County of Shanxi Province* in 1644, and in *The Annals of Jianggang in Jilin's Changbai Mountain* at the end of the Qing Dynasty in China. KD was reported in 1907 according to some historical data. At that time, some farmers migrated from Liaoning Province to Keshan County in Heilongjiang Province to reclaim the wastelands. After living there for two to three years, the inhabitants began suffering from a disease which had similar symptoms with KD. Above-mentioned facts proved that Chinese people had a long history in the understanding of endemic diseases. However, the scientific understanding and control of the endemic diseases did not occur until the modern times.

Before P.R. China was founded, although a few researchers had done a small number of population surveys or described individual cases on some endemic diseases, few scientific experiments were carried out, except a study of Dr. Liande Wu on the transmission route of plague from 1910 to 1931. Dr. Wu found that the marmot was the intermediate host of plague, and proposed "pneumonic plague" theory. Dr. Liande Wu made historic contributions for plague control (Fig. 1.10). From 1910 to 1911, plague outbroke in the northeast of China. At that time, Russia and Japan once claimed monopoly power on epidemic prevention. The excuse was to protect their emigrants. Compelled by the situation, Chinese government designated Dr. Liande Wu, who was Vice-Director of the Imperial Army Medical College, as general medical officer. As soon as Dr. Liande Wu arrived in Harbin city which was the worst region involved, he took decisive measures like "strengthen prevention, control the traffic, isolate the infected areas, establish medical institutions, receive patients, burn corpses of the dead, and others". After six months of efforts, the epidemic was extinguished. From 1940 to 1942, Xunyuan Yao and Yongzheng Yao made some useful explorations on endemic goiter prevention (Fig. 1.11). They performed investigations on endemic goiter in 37 counties in Yunnan Province. On the basis of this survey, in the mid-1940s, a study in the salt mines of Pinglang of Yunnan Province was conducted in order to control the endemic goiter by using iodized salt, which was the beginning of large-scale prevention on IDD. In addition, during 1930s and 1940s, some Japanese medical experts in the former South

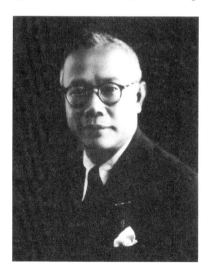

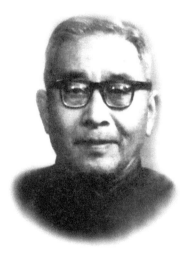

Fig. 1.10　Dr. Liande Wu (1879-1960) Known as the "Plague Fighter" in China and even in the world.

Fig. 1.11　Dr. Yongzheng Yao, who was the first scientist to control the endemic goiter by using iodized salt in China.

Manchuria Medical College located in Shenyang City of Liaoning Province undertook the research on etiology of Keshan disease and Kashin-Beck disease in order for Japan to annex the northeast of China. In general, the situation of endemic disease in China was in "out of control" status. Preventive measures were rarely taken, and endemic diseases became the most serious public health problem that threatened the people's health and life in old China. According to documents, in the first half of the 20th century, there were six plague pandemics, spreading over 20 provinces and autonomous regions, in which 1.15 million inhabitants were involved and 1.02 million inhabitants died. Schistosomiasis and KSD were once rampantly prevalent in hundreds of counties, which destroyed many villages and families. The harms resulting from KBD, IDD and endemic fluorosis were too appalling, which aggravated the suffering of Chinese people at that time. No reliable statistic data were found about the endemic diseases in the old China.

After the founding of P. R. China, the Chinese government has always emphasized great importance to the prevention and control of endemic diseases. Chairman Mao Zedong who was also the Chairman of the Central Committee of the Communist Party of China personally supervised the nationwide schistosomiasis control, and wrote the famous poetry "Get away, pest!" (Fig. 1.12). Premier Zhou Enlai directly arranged the work on its control and designated medical stuffs and

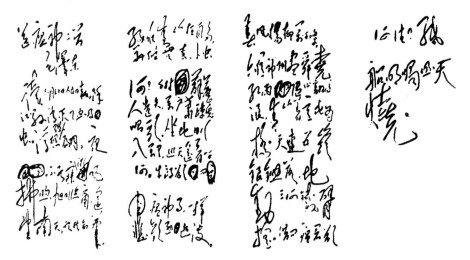

Fig. 1.12 President Mao Zedong wrote the poetry "Get away, Pest!" in 1958 when he knew schistosomiasis had been wiped out in Yujiang county, Jiangxi province.

researchers to severely affected areas. During the reform and opening-up period since 1978, top leader Deng Xiaoping wrote the glorious inscription "Control endemic diseases for the benefits of the people" (Fig. 1.13). Chinese government leaders like Jiang Zemin, Hu Jintao and Xi Jinping, also made many important instructions for the endemic disease control. They were very concerned about the health of the inhabitants in endemic disease areas. When P. R. China was established, the state government organized medical specialists to investigate and control plague, schistosomiasis, KD, KBD and brucellosis. In 1955, Chairman Mao Zedong proposed to establish the state leading group for schistosomiasis prevention and control. In 1956, "National Program for Agricultural Development" was developed under the leadership of Chairman Mao Zedong, which clearly proposed the objectives of eliminating schistosomiasis and plague, to actively control KD, KBD and endemic goiter. In 1957, the State Council issued a program on the elimination of schistosomiasis. In 1960, the state leading group for the prevention and control of the endemic diseases prevalent in northern China was established, and relevant leading groups and specialized institutions were also set up in succession at the provincial level in the whole country. In 1981, with the approval of the CPC Central Committee,

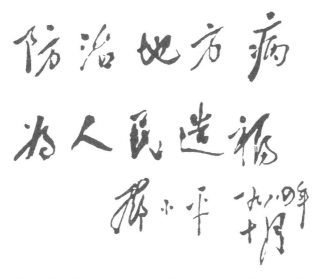

Fig. 1.13 The inscription written by the national leader Deng Xiaoping, means "controlling endemic disease for the benefits of people".

the function of the state leading group for the prevention and control of endemic diseases in northern China was expanded to the whole country, renamed as the state leading group for the endemic disease prevention and control. The members of the Political Bureau of the CPC Central Committee or candidate members, such as Lanfu Wu, Xilian Chen and Desheng Li were appointed as leaders of the group respectively (Fig. 1.15). In 1986, the Bureau for Endemic Disease Control was established in the Ministry of Health to replace the State Leading Group for the Endemic Disease Prevention and Control. In the meantime, the Chinese Center for Endemic Disease Control and Research and the National Base for Plague and Brucellosis Control was established (Fig. 1.14). In 1998, together with parasitic diseases, the management of endemic diseases control was transferred to the Department for Disease Prevention and Control in the Ministry of Health. In 2004, the management of the endemic disease control was separated from the parasitic diseases, and incorporated into the Division for Rural Water and Toilet Improvement in the National Office of Patriotic

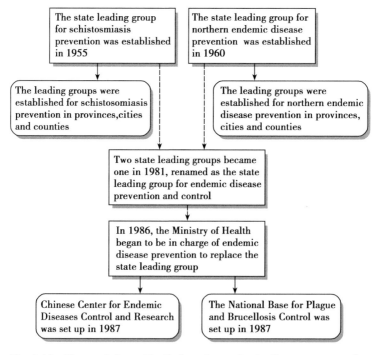

Fig. 1.14　The evolution of institutions for endemic diseases prevention and control in China

Health Campaign Committee. In 2006, with the personnel expansion of the Department for Disease Prevention and Control in the Ministry of Health, the Office for Endemic Disease Control and Prevention was established, which was in charge of the management of national endemic disease control. From the beginning of the 21st century, under the close attention of the Chinese government, the Ministry of Health drew up the National Plan for Key Endemic Diseases Prevention and Control from 2004 to 2010, and the National "Twelfth-Five Year" Plan for all the Endemic Diseases Prevention and Control. By the two plans, the project of central government subsidies to local public health special fund for endemic disease control and the project of the national safe drinking water provided for rural residents were implemented. 62 billion RMB was invested, and amazing progresses had been achieved for endemic disease control.

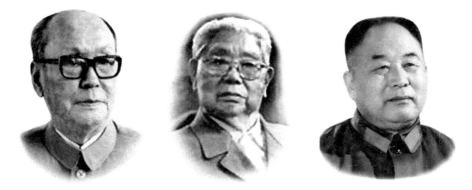

Fig. 1.15 The leaders of the group for endemic disease prevention in China. Right: Lanfun Wu (1960-1988); Middle: Xilian Chen (1915-1999); Right: Desheng Li (1916-2011).

During the fight with the endemic diseases for nearly half a century, China invested a lot of human and material resources, establishing a series of administrative organizations and professional institutions from national to local levels for endemic disease control and prevention. The Ministry of Health has organized multi-unit and cross-disciplinary scientific investigation for many times, such as the investigation led by Professor Weihan Yu on KD in Chuxiong County of Yunnan Province, KBD investigation led by Professor Jianbo Yang in Yongshou County of Shaanxi Province, and the pilot control project for the coal-burning type fluorosis in Three Gorges areas which was carried out by the Chinese Center for Endemic Disease Control and

Prevention and the Chinese Academy of Preventive Medicine. National Sci & Tech projects and Supporting Programs for the endemic disease research were continuously set up. China also cooperated effectively with international organizations on endemic disease control and research. The endemic diseases were controlled on a large scale, especially in recent years, due to a large amount of the central government funds investment such as transfer payments by the central government and the state's key project for health care reform. And remarkable achievements have been obtained. First, the research on etiology, epidemiological investigations, surveillance and preventive measures have reached the world's advanced level; second, the incidence of endemic diseases is significantly decreased nationwide. At present, no acute KD case occurs, KBD trend is completely under control in the eastern region, IDD status is at the elimination level, and disabled skeletal fluorosis is almost controlled.

The achievements on controlling the endemic diseases should be attributed to the leadership of the Chinese government, close cooperation among relevant departments, and active participation of inhabitants living in the endemic disease areas. We should never forget the old scientists, such as Professor Liande Wu, Weihan Yu, Shoubai Mao, Xianyi Zhu, Jianbo Yang, Shuli Ji, Shichen Wang, Jianan Tan, Jianqun Li, Shouren Cao and so on. They made important contributions to the endemic disease research and control in China.

1.6 Achievements for the Endemic Disease Control in China

In order to consolidate the achievements on the endemic disease control, establish long-term working mechanism to adapt to the economic and social development and completely eliminate the hazards of endemic diseases, through a Project for Endemic Disease Control from Key Public Health Service Projects, the central government invested nearly one billion RMB in the mid-western regions for the control and prevention of endemic diseases from 2011 to 2015. The project included surveillance, implementation of preventive measures, patient treatment, health education and personnel training as well as capacity building of the organizations for endemic

disease control. In order to implement the Twelfth Five-Year Plan for the residents'
drinking water safety in rural areas, the central government invested 155 billion RMB
to construct safety drinking water projects in high-fluorine and high-arsenic areas and
other areas where drinking water is not safe. The other government departments in
agriculture, forestry and poverty alleviation implemented many comprehensive
measures for the endemic disease control, consequently improving the ecological
environment and accelerating the control of endemic diseases in China.

1. 6. 1   Iodine Deficiency Disorders

Since 2010, no new cases of endemic cretinism were found in China. By the end of
2012, all of surveillance indicators had reached the standard required for IDD
elimination, such as coverage rate of qualified iodized salt, goiter rate of children
aged 8-10, median of urinary iodine and the ratio of urinary iodine being less than
50mg/L of children aged 8-10 and others. At present, IDD has already been at the
level of sustained elimination in China, the overall level of iodine nutrition is
appropriate for the entire Chinese population, and 96.4% of all counties in China
have achieved the goal for IDD sustained elimination. More than 95% of counties in
each province, except Tibet, Xinjiang and Qinghai, have reached the goal for IDD
sustained elimination. In Tibet only 86.5% of counties have reached the goal. In
high iodine drinking water areas, no-iodized salt was supplied for controlling the
diseases related to high iodine exposure, such as goiter, hypothyroidism,
autoimmune thyroid diseases etc., covering about 82% of the counties exposed to
high iodine in drinking water by 2012. In the high iodine areas of Beijing and Inner
Mongolia, water-improvement measures have been taken to secure drinking water
safety and the iodine content in drinking water has been reduced to the national
standard (<100mg/L).

1. 6. 2   Endemic Fluorosis

1. 6. 2. 1   *Drinking Water Type Fluorosis*
In endemic areas of drinking water type fluorosis, detectable rate of children dental
fluorosis has declined year by year, and the downward trends have also been shown
in the detectable rates of clinical skeletal fluorosis and X-ray skeletal fluorosis. In

2010, new drinking water projects in 72.3 thousand villages were built in fluorosis areas, and the overall rate of water quality improvement was 83. 08%. In severely affected areas, the quality of drinking water in 7. 8 thousand villages had been improved, and the improvement rate of water quality reached 92. 15%. The improvement rate of water quality in the 25. 3 thousand villages in moderate areas reached 88. 76%. Compared with the surveyed result in 2005, the overall rate of water quality improvement was increased by 38. 38% in 2010. Normal operation rate of drinking water projects was 92. 78% in all the affected areas. From the survey result of 2010, detectable rate of dental fluorosis of children aged 8-12 reached 25. 03% in improved water villages, and dental fluorosis index was 0. 53 which belonged to edge popular. However, it had already reached the standard for endemic fluorosis control. By the end of 2012, the overall rate of water quality improvement rate was 82. 27%. The drinking water quality of all waterworks in Beijing, Fujian, Hubei, Hunan, Guangdong, Tibet and Chongqing had totally reached the water quality improvement standard (Fluoride<1. 2mg/L). The normal usage rate of these drinking water projects to decrease fluoride in China was about 85%, except Hubei Province (74.45%), and all the other provinces were over 95%.

1. 6. 2. 2   Coal-burning Type Endemic Fluorosis

In the endemic areas of coal-burning type fluorosis, detectable rate of dental fluorosis of children aged 8-12 has been sharply decreased, and in some provinces it has dropped to the controlled level. Among 8.23 million households, 7.45 million had improved stoves with chimney before 2010 through the support of the central government, reaching the rate of 90. 61%. And 7. 06 million households could correctly use these improved stoves, correct usage rate reaching 94. 74%, and benefiting 29.39 million inhabitants. During 2011-2012, the stoves with chimneys in 720 thousand households were introduced, accounting for 8. 77 % of all households in the affected areas. And 710 thousand households could use them correctly, the correct usage rate reaching about 98.33% and benefiting 3.02 million inhabitants. By the end of 2012, a total of 8.16 million stoves had been improved. The rate of improved stoves was about 99.38%, the correct usage rate was about 95.06%, and the benefited population was 32.41 million, accounting for 96.03% of the whole population in the coal-burning type fluorosis areas. Among the surveyed provinces, the rate of improved stoves reached 100% in Beijing, Shanxi, Liaoning, Jiangxi, Henan and Chongqing, and other provinces were all more than 95%. Correct usage rates of improved stoves were all over 95%, except Shanxi, Hubei and Chongqing. In 2012, the rate of knowledge awareness about the coal-buring type fluorosis prevention and control was between 85.0% and 92.4% among housewives.

1.6.2.3 Drinking Brick-tea Type Fluorosis

By the end of 2012, the endemic areas of drinking brick-tea type fluorosis in China had been basically ascertained, and the standard for the fluorine content in brick tea had been established. At present, annual sales of brick tea were about 24,400 tons in drinking brick-tea type fluorosis areas, and the sales of brick tea with qualified fluorine content were 2,163 tons, accounting for 8.87% of the total sales. Especially, the sale ratio of brick tea with qualified fluorine content was higher in Ningxia, which was about 58%, followed by 19.44% in Xinjiang.

1.6.3 Endemic arsenicosis

1.6.3.1 Drinking Water Type Arsenicosis

In the endemic areas of drinking water type arsenicosis, the rate of improved water has been continuously increased, and the prevalence of arsenicosis is relatively stable after water improvement. During 2009-2012, no new cases of arsenicosis were identified, so were no new cases of skin cancer in these surveillance villages. By the end of 2012, a total of 828 villages had improved the quality of drinking water in drinking water type arsenicosis areas for local people to drink safe lower-arsenic water through building new waterworks, and the rate of improved water was about 93.56%. The waterworks in 782 villages were normally operated, accounting for 94.44% of all surveyed villages, which benefited population 520 thousand, accounting for 82.84% of all inhabitants living in those arsenicosis areas. In high-arsenic areas, 828 villages had improved the quality of drinking water, and the rate of improved water was about 86.25%. The waterworks in 1,628 villages were in normal operation, accounting for 93.67%, which benefited 1.14 million inhabitants, accounting for 79.78% of all the inhabitants in the affected areas.

1.6.3.2 Coal-burning Type Arsenicosis

Coal-burning type arsenicosis only occurs in China, and only in Guizhou and Shanxi provinces of western China. Before 2007, measures of improved stoves with chimney had been completely taken to control arsenicosis, covering 37 million households. In 2010, the correct usage rate of improved stoves was about 92.23%. Based on the survey data from 2006 to 2010, no new cases were identified, and the prevalence of arsenicosis was stable.

1.6.4 Kashin-Beck Disease

Since 1990, KBD has been continuously monitored for 25 years. The results show that the prevalence of KBD has been effectively controlled along with the rapid development of economy, society and people's quality of life as well as the implementation of comprehensive preventive measures. Since 2000, in eastern and central regions of China (Heilongjiang, Jilin, Liaoning, Shandong, Shanxi, Hebei and Henan provinces), the prevalence of children KBD has been continuously at the control level, and it has also declined in the western regions year by year (Inner Mongolia, Shanxi, Gansu, Sichuan, Tibet and Qinghai provinces). From the surveillance data of 13 provinces in 2014, the clinical detectable rate of children KBD was 0.01%, and the X-ray positive detectable rate was only 0.17%. By the end of 2015, China had achieved the goal of basically eliminating KBD, which means that KBD in more than 90% of the affected areas have been removed.

1.6.5 Keshan Disease

At present, acute KD has not been found for more than 20 years in China, and subacute KD has not been detected for nearly 10 years. The nationwide prevalence is generally at the level of control. Therefore, it appears a stable and controlled trend. From the surveillance result of 2010, the total detectable rate of KD in these affected areas was 2.2%. Among them, the latent type KD accounted for 1.7%, the chronic type KD was only 0.5%, and the incidence of KD was obviously decreased as compared with the surveillance results of 2005 (total detectable rate was 4.1%, and latent type and chronic type KD were 3.5% and 0.6% respectively). By the end of 2012, a total of 221 counties in 11 provinces out of 16 provinces with KD areas had been assessed in order to find out the progress of KD control. Among them, 213 counties reached the national control standard, up to the rate of 96.4%. From 2011 to 2015, 2,663 KD patients were treated, and 6.93 million inhabitants were supplemented with selenium through projects funded by the central government.

1.7　The Strategy for Endemic Disease Control and Prevention in China

The occurrence of endemic disease is related to natural ecological factors and the distribution of elements in the special environment, which are the characteristics of endemic formation. This determines that the endemic disease control and prevention is long-term, arduous and complex. Because it is difficult to eliminate such causative factors, once the control and prevention becomes slack, the incidence rate will rebound. More importantly, endemic occurrence is due to biogeochemical factors or unhealthy behavior lifestyle. Therefore, in order to continuously consolidate the results of prevention to avoid reoccurrence, we should establish a long-term preventive working mechanism in the endemic disease areas where comprehensive prevention and control measures have already been implemented.

Currently, certain endemic diseases are still prevalent in some areas of China. Endemic diseases are still public health problems in rural area of China, and they are also important diseases that need long-term control and prevention in the future. Western provinces are key regions for the endemic diseases prevention. So far, China has three provinces in the western region which have not eliminated IDD. KBD is mainly distributed in the Tibetan Plateau, where serious X-ray changes of KBD in children can still be detected in some villages. There are still young chronic cases of KD in the western areas of China. Similarly, other endemic diseases are mostly concentrated in the western region of China, such as coal-burning fluorosis, coal-burning arsenicosis, and brick-tea fluorosis. Therefore, focus should be put on western China for endemic disease control. In addition, in both the western and central regions, the prevention tasks for drinking water type fluorosis are still arduous. We should not only improve the quality of drinking water, but manage the waterworks as well, to fully use the water improvement projects and further to control drinking water type fluorosis. Achieving this goal still needs a tremendous effort.

Therefore, China's endemic disease prevention strategy is that a sustainable mechanism for endemic disease elimination should be established. The measures include: (1) Keeping prevention organizations for endemic disease, and stabilizing research teams for endemic disease; (2) Strengthening surveillance, establishing the national information management systems of endemic diseases to master the dynamic trend, and implementing sound prevention plans; (3) Carrying out scientific research, to reveal the etiology and pathogenesis of endemic diseases, and to utilize advanced techniques in time for the scientific control of endemic diseases; (4) Emphasizing health education, to popularize the knowledge of endemic disease control and prevention, and to guide the residents living in the endemic disease areas to participate in and cooperate with the national preventive measures for endemic disease control.

In formulating the endemic disease prevention strategies, based on the understanding of endemic etiology and characteristics, we must uphold the following five principles:

1.7.1　Adhere to the Principle that Endemic Disease is still the Major Disease Endangering the Health of Rural Residents in China

This is determined by the feature of etiology and pathogenesis of Chinese endemic diseases. At present, endemic diseases are popular to varying degrees in 31 Chinese provinces, autonomous regions and municipalities. Serious diseases are mainly concentrated in western China, mostly in impoverished, rural, remote and ethnic minority areas. Moreover, the local natural environment is unlikely to be changed. Once the control and prevention become slack, the incidence rate will rebound. Endemic diseases not only seriously harm the health of the people, but also hinder the economic development of the endemic disease areas. It is one of important reasons for local residents poverty caused by illness or return-to-poverty by illness. Therefore, the Chinese government has always put endemic and infectious diseases together as prominent issues that seriously affect the health status of rural residents in China.

1.7.2 Adhere to the Working Mechanism "Government Leadership, Department Cooperation and Masses to Participate in" for the Endemic Disease Control

This is determined by the characteristics of the preventive measures of endemic diseases. The management of endemic diseases belongs to the health sector, but most of the relevant preventive measures are taken by other departments. For example, water improvement, stove improvement, salt iodization, changing grain and relocation do not belong to the scope of responsibilities of the health sector. Thus, the health sector hasn't the right and the power to carry out the relevant work. Therefore, relevant departments must closely cooperate for the endemic disease control and prevention. Otherwise, the health sector alone will not be able to implement necessary measures to achieve the goal in endemic disease control and prevention. Thus, the health sector should abandon the old thinking and habits that implement all the measures alone in endemic disease control and prevention, recognizes its own responsibilities, conducts investigation and research on endemic diseases, provides scientific and effective control measures, develops various endemic health standards, and formulates control plans and strategies. Meanwhile, the health sector should take the initiative to coordinate relevant departments to implement control measures and to clarify their responsibilities through administrative regulations or systems. Obviously, the coordination of these departments is inseparable from the organization and leadership of the government. The successful experience of China for the endemic disease control shows that the government should attach great importance to the control and prevention of endemic diseases, makes it become a part of the government's function. In 1960, the Central Government Leading Group of the Northern Endemic Disease Control was established (in 1981, the work was extended to the whole country, renamed the National Leading Group of Endemic Disease Control), and played a major role on the prevention and control of endemic diseases. Based on the characteristics of endemic disease prevention measures and the current condition, leading organizations should be established at all levels for endemic disease prevention. Implementing measures to control endemic diseases can not be separated from the active participation of the masses. For example, in the endemic areas of coal-burning fluorosis, some residents do not use the government-issued defluoridation stoves. They are accustomed to using the open burning stoves, and even sell out the defluoridation stoves. Some residents do not take the initiative to repair the damaged defluoridation stoves, and they think it is the obligation of the government. Similar situations exist in other endemic diseases. Therefore, in order to achieve the goal of broad participation of residents for the endemic disease control and prevention, we must further strengthen health education and health promotion, and actively explore scientific and effective health education contents and measures. In the areas where conditions permit, we should mobilize residents and government officers to work together for endemic disease control.

1. 7. 3　Adhere to the Principle of "Based on Prevention, Taking into account the Treatment" for the Endemic Disease Control

This is determined by the clinical characteristics of endemic diseases, which can be prevented but can not be cured. Although most endemic diseases (excluding natural foci endemic diseases) are not like some infectious diseases that spread in a short period of time and cause death, the outcomes of some endemic diseases are very serious and cause severe disability (for example, degree II KBD, skeletal fluorosis and cretinism) and even death (such as acute type, subacute type and late stage chronic KD patients, and severe endemic arsenicosis patients). For endemic disease patients who survive disabilities, they not only lose the ability to work, but also cannot take care of themselves, so their "quality of life" is poor. Therefore, we have always insisted on principle "prevention first" for endemic disease control. However, we can not only emphasize "prevention first" and completely ignore the treatment of endemic diseases. During 1950s and 1960s, acute and subacute type KD outbroke and needed emergency treatment. Although this situation no longer exists currently, the number of endemic disease patients is mainly due to old patients' accumulation for many years. The numbers of skeletal fluorosis patients of drinking water type and coal-burning type are 1. 34 million and 1.95 million respectively; adult KBD patients have reached 640 thousand; and there are nearly 40 thousand latent and chronic KD patients. If these patients are not treated adequately in time, their disease condition will become increasingly worse, and brings great suffering and economic burden to the patients and their family. Therefore, the government has the responsibility to treat them. Moreover, this work can help the government carry out the prevention of endemic diseases. Otherwise, residents in endemic disease areas will not take the initiative for long-term efforts to cooperate with local government or CDC for the endemic disease control. Therefore, we must correctly handle the relationship between endemic disease prevention and treatment. It is necessary to focus on improving the precaution of endemic disease, and make therapeutics simultaneously. This conforms to the principle of "truly based on prevention, taking into account the treatment".

1.7.4 Adhere to the Principle of "To give the Priority to the Key Endemic Area, Key Endemic Disease, and Key Population"

This is determined by the epidemiological characteristics. In China, endemic diseases are distributed in widespread areas, affecting a large population. Only in the key endemic areas the diseases are severe, and only in key population the diseases show the serious threat. In the case of fund shortage for arduous task of prevention and treatment, the implementation of control measures and the arrangement of preventive projects should be in accordance with "the priority of serious patients" and "easy things first". The endemic disease surveillance and survey data indicated: (1) Western regions in China should be the focus areas with the priority for endemic disease control; (2) Compared with the situation in 1970s and 1980s, the focus on the prevention and treatment of endemic diseases has changed. Currently, IDD and endemic fluorosis have become main targets; (3) The key population of the endemic disease prevention and treatment are fetuses, children, women of childbearing age, malnourished people, and so on.

1.7.5 Adhere to the Principle of "Research Serves the Prevention and Treatment of Endemic Diseases"

This is determined by the core work of the endemic disease control. Over the years, the working principles of endemic disease control that adhere to the work-centered and research-based prevention and treatment and research serving endemic disease prevention have resulted in a huge effect to control endemic diseases, especially KD and KBD. The following is a summary of the hot issues or topics related to endemic disease control: (1) IDD:1) Pathogenesis of iodine deficiency disease at molecular level, mainly in brain damage due to different degrees of iodine deficiency during brain development, and other factors involved in this process; 2) Harmful effects of high iodine levels on the human body and its pathogenesis. (2) Endemic fluorosis:1) Pathogenesis of endemic fluorosis, especially epidemiological and pathogenesis studies of non-bone tissues; 2) Prevention and treatment for different types of endemic fluorosis; 3) Prevention and treatment measures for grade II or III skeletal fluorosis. (3) endemic arsenicosis:1) Pathogenesis of endemic arsenic poisoning, especially on pathogenesis for hazards of long-term arsenic exposure, with priorities for visceral tumors, cardiovascular diseases and genetic toxicity; 2) Research on effective drugs for the treatment of endemic arsenicosis; 3) Water arsenic hygiene standards and the classification criteria of disease regions in Chinese mainland. (4) KBD:1) Research on etiology and pathogenesis of KBD; 2) Research on the treatment of adult KBD. (5) KD: 1) Research on etiology and pathogenesis research of KD; 2) Specific diagnostic methods of KD.

1.8　The Experience for Endemic Disease Control and Prevention in China

After sixty years of scientific prevention and control of endemic diseases, China has made great achievements and accumulated valuable experiences that are summarized as follows.

1.8.1　To Strengthen Government Leadership is a Key to do a Good Job in the Prevention and Control of Endemic Diseases

In the initial period of P. R. China, the Central Committee of the Communist Party of China saw the prevention and control of endemic diseases as an important political task. The older generation of the national leaders, including Mao Zedong, Zhou Enlai, Deng Xiaoping, et al., wrote inscriptions in order to promote the implementation of preventive measures for endemic disease prevention and control. In 1955, the Chinese southern leading group for schistosomiasis prevention and control was founded, and in 1960 the Chinese northern leading group for endemic disease control and prevention was established. These two leading groups merged into one as the national leading group for endemic disease prevention and control in 1981. The leading group was responsible for the formulation of strategies and plans, organizing professional teams, and the enhancement of legal management, coordinating or organizing relevant deparments to implennent the measures in the control of endemic diseases. After 1986, the Endemic Disease Prevention and Control Bureau, the Ministry of Health (later replaced by Disease Control Bureau) and the leading groups at provincial levels effectively guided the practice of endemic disease prevention and control in China.

1. 8. 2　Close Cooperation among the Relevant Departments is an Effective and Fundamental Measure to Carry out Prevention and Control of Endemic Diseases

The implementation of the prevention and control measures for endemic diseases involves lots of regions and departments, and thus must be done by the relevant departments collaboratively in accordance with their respective divisional functions and duties. Over the past 60 years, the relevant departments in China have actively played crucial role in the prevention and control of endemic diseases. The waterworks department implemented water-improving measures with the priority in endemic areas of fluorosis and arsenicosis. The salt industry department improved the iodized salt supply and market network, and popularized the iodized salt for IDD prevention. The forestry department implemented the project of returning farmland to forests and grassland with the priority in KBD areas. The development and reform department gave top priority to the endemic disease areas when the construction projects conducive to the comprehensive measures of the endemic disease areas were considered promoting the social and economic development of these areas. The financial department increased the investment for the endemic disease prevention and control year by year.

1. 8. 3　Combination with Poverty Alleviation is the Basic Guideline to be followed in the Prevention and Control of Endemic Diseases

Severe endemic areas are mainly distributed in the remote, poor, and ethnic minority regions. The prevalence of endemic diseases in these regions results in a vicious circle of "illness due to poverty and poverty due to illness", highlighting an important public health problem in local regions. After the Third Plenary Session of the 11th Central Committee of the CPC, most rural areas in China successfully got rid of poverty, as a result the prevalence of KD and KBD was basically controlled. Previous practice demonstrated that the policy of combining the prevention and treatment of diseases together with poverty alleviation played a decisive role in breaking the vicious cycle of poverty and illness.

1.8.4 To Strengthen the Legal System Development and insist on the Law-based Prevention and Control are the Powerful Means to Ensure the Smooth Progress of Endemic Disease Prevention and Control

In order to ensure that the prevention and control of endemic diseases can be carried out scientifically, the national and local governments as well as relevant departments developed and published a series of laws and regulations, including *The management regulations of iodized salt to eliminate the hazard of IDD* issued by the State Council. With the aim to guide the surveillance and control of endemic diseases scientifically, an endemic disease standard system has been established, including 1) the diagnostic criteria of endemic diseases; 2) the delimitation and classification of endemic diseases; 3) the assessment of therapeutic principles and effects of endemic diseases; 4) the standard of implementing measures for the prevention and control of endemic diseases; 5) the standard for endemic disease control and elimination; 6) the standards for endemic disease laboratory. By the end of 2012, a total of 69 standards, including 34 national standards and 35 industrial standards, were formulated or revised by the Standard Committee of Endemic Diseases. Fifty-seven standards were promulgated, including 27 national standards and 30 industrial standards. The issue of these regulations and technical specifications has effectively ensured the smooth and well-regulated operation for endemic disease prevention and control, and promoted the process of endemic disease elimination.

1. 8. 5 To Strengthen the Capacity Building of the Prevention and Control Institutions is the Organizational Guarantee to carry out the Control and Research Activities of Endemic Diseases

Our professional institutions and teams of endemic disease prevention and control began to be built at the early stage of P. R. China, and were then gradually developed in the fight against the endemic diseases. At the stage of high incidence of endemic diseases, lots of researchers went to endemic areas to perform investigations, implement preventive measures, treat patients, and do scientific research. They tackled many difficulties and got lots of important data on scientific research of etiology, pathogenesis, control measures, and treatment methods.

1. 8. 6 To Improve the Surveillance System is the Basis for Scientific Evaluation and Adjustment of Prevention and Control Strategies for Endemic Diseases

The investigation of endemic disease prevalence during the pandemic period laid groundwork for the establishment of the endemic disease surveillance system. In 1989, the Endemic Disease Control Division under the Ministry of Health issued *Notification on the establishment of the national endemic disease surveillance sites*, which marked the initial establishment of endemic disease surveillance system. This system was gradually improved in the later practice. From 2007 to 2009, the surveillance program was revised, and the original focus on key sites surveillance was changed to sampling surveillance nationwide. In 2012, the surveillance programs were further revised. At present, the endemic disease surveillance system characterized by high sensitivity and wide coverage has been basically formed, which has strengthened the surveillance itself in combination with interventions, providing scientific basis for the timely evaluation and adjustment of prevention and control strategies. In recent years, on the basis of China's improved endemic surveillance system, information management systems of IDD has been established, and thousands of data access points nationwide gave access to a data capacity of a million records or more per year, which has greatly speeded up information transmission and improved the ability in analyzing the control effect on endemic diseases.

1. 8. 7 Promoting Extensive Health Eeducation is the Basis for Mobilizing the General Public to Actively Participate in the Endemic Disease Prevention and Control

For many years, by means of such measures as mass media and interpersonal communication, professional institutions and related departments at all levels carried out plentiful and various forms of health education activities, which had made knowledge of endemic disease prevention and control known to every family and deep into people's heart, and further strengthened the disease prevention awareness and promoted the formation of healthy behavior and good life style of people. In particular, "The publicity day for IDD prevention" activity in May 15th every year has become a model for health education of endemic diseases, playing an important role in the prevention and control of IDD. In recent years, through the implementation of the health education of the central subsidy from major public health projects, the residents in endemic areas have become aware of the hazards of endemic diseases and their old living style has been transformed.

1. 8. 8 To Strengthen the International Cooperation is the Technical Support to Promote the Development of Endemic Disease Prevention and Control

Since the mid-1980s, Chinese government has strengthened the cooperation and communication with the World Health Organization (WHO), the United Nations International Children's Emergency Fund (UNICEF), and other international organizations in the field of endemic disease prevention and control. In more than 20 years, dozens of cooperation projects have been finished.

In 1985, the prevention and treatment of KBD in China was included into the UNICEF cooperation project, including many research projects. For example, the case-control investigation of KBD was finished in 1990, the observation of VC and selenium effect on KBD prevention and treatment was finished in 1991, and the observation of grain drying effect on the prevention and control of KBD was finished at the beginning of 1994. From 1989 to 1991, as partnership with the WHO, historical data collection, sorting, summarizing, translation, and communication on the etiological and epidemiological studies of KBD were undertaken.

In 1993, the Ministry of Health and the UNICEF launched an international cooperation program to eliminate IDD. The first and second cycle of cooperation was committed to promoting the implementation of universal salt iodization (USI) strategy, equipping laboratory instruments for IDD surveillance, and personnel training on cooperative projects. From 2001 to 2005, it was decided to strengthen the implementation of key interventions in the major western and coastal provinces in the third cycle of cooperative projects between the Ministry of Health and the UNICEF. The purpose of this project was to eliminate the hazard of IDD, to correct women's and children's iodine nutrition deficiency, and to improve the health level. The adopted strategies mainly included social mobilization, providing better iodized salt production and sales network, carrying out health education and promotion activities, and supporting China's IDD surveillance, and so on. After 2006, focusing on major problems of the prevention and control of IDD in China, many projects were financed including the investigation of the high-risk areas of IDD, the investigation of iodine nutrition in the coastal areas, the investigation of iodine nutrition in pregnant women, and the prevention and control strategies of high iodine areas.

From 2002, the Ministry of Health and the UNICEF launched the project to mitigate the risk of arsenic poisoning. In 2002, screening for high arsenic water was conducted in relevant provinces. At the same time, the development of half quantitative reagent kit for high arsenic water was supported. By 2006, the water arsenic screening work had been finished, and the distribution of high arsenic in drinking water in China was basically clarified. Then based on the national high arsenic water screening results, the GIS system of high arsenic areas was established to serve for the prevention and control of the endemic arsenicosis in China. Thanks to the major work of the prevention and control of endemic arsenicosis in China, activities such as knowledge popularization, personnel training, laboratory capacity building, and the compilation of pictorial manual for endemic diseases diagnosis were developed.

Above-mentioned cooperation projects have effectively promoted the prevention and control of endemic diseases in China, and expanded the international influence of China in the field of endemic disease prevention and control.

Further Reading

1. SUN Dian-jun. Endemiology. Beijing: People's Medical Publishing House.2011.

2. Qian Xin-zhong. Endemiology-The Medical Encyclopedia of China. Shanghai: Shanghai Science and Technology Prss.1983.

3. John M. Last. A Dictionary of Epidemiology. Fourth Edition. Oxford Univeersity Press. 2001.

4. YangJianbo.The study on the Etiology of Kashin-Beck Disease. Harbin: Heilongjiang Science and Technology Press. 1998.

5. Yu Wei-han. Chinese Keshan Disease. Harbin: Heilongjiang Science and Technology Press. 2003.

6. Endemic Disease Control, Chinese Center for Disease Control and Prevention. Handbook of Iodine Deficiency Disorders Prevention and Control. Beijing: People's Medical Publishing House.2007.

7. SUN Dian-jun. Surveillance of Iodine Deficiency Disorders in China,2011. Beijing: People's Medical Publishing House.2014.

8. SUN Dian-jun. Handbook of Endemic Fluorosis Prevention and Control. Beijing: People's Medical Publishing House.2012.

9. SUN Dian-jun. Pictorial Manual for Endemic Arsenicosis Diagnosis. Beijing: People's Medical Publishing House.2015.

10. SUN Dian-jun. Handbook of Kaschin-Beck Disease Prevention and Control. Beijing: People's Medical Publishing House.2016.

11. World Health Organization. Guidelines for Drinking-water Quality. Third Edition. 2004.

12. Tony Appelo. Arsenic in Groundwater-A World Problem. Netherlands National Committee-International Association of Hydrogeologists (NNC-IAH). 2006.

13. Pei Hanhua, Liang Shuxiong, Ning Lianyuan. The investigation to enrichment pattern of groundwater arsenic and its forming cause in Datong Basin. Hydro geological engineering geology.2005,32(4):65-69.

14. Sun Dianjun.Sorting and understanding of the major prevention and control problems for key endemic diseases in China . Chinese Journal of Endemiology.2014,33(2):59-62.

15. SUN Dian-jun. Sorting and understanding of the major research problems for key endemic diseases in China.Chinese Journal of Endemiology.2013,32:1-5.

16. Sun Dianjun.Prospect of the endemic disease control in China.Chinese Journal of Endemiology. 2009,28(1):3-6.

17. Wang Maowu,Sun Dianjun.Six principles for endemic disease control and prevention. Chinese Journal of Endemiology.2004,23(5):397-399.

18. Sun Dianjun, Shen Hongmei, Wei Honglian. The historical process, experience and prospect of endemic disease surveillance in China.Chinese Journal of Endemiology.2009,28(2):123-125.

19. Sun Dianjun, Wei Honglian, Shen Hongmei, et al. Fifty years of endemic disease control and prevention in China. Chinese Journal of Endemiology.2003,22(2):20-23.

20. Sun Dianjun.Interpreting the 60-year experience of endemic disease control and prevention in China. Chinese Journal of Endemiology. 2013,32(6):595-598.

21. Sun Dianjun, Shen Hongmei, Li Xun,et al. Review of the 11th Five-Year period and Prospect of the 12th Five-Year period for the control and prevention of key endemic diseases in China. Chinese Journal of Endemiology. 2012, 31(5):473-475.

22. Lei Zhenglong, Yan Jun, Zhang Shubin, et al. Situation and major tasks for the control and prevention of key endemic diseases. Chinese Journal of Endemiology. 2014,33(5):475-478.

Chapter 2

Iodine Deficiency Disorders (IDD)

Shoujun Liu, Ming Li, Lijun Fan, Peng Liu, Fangang Meng, Xiaohui Su, and Zhaojun Zhang

Abstract

Iodine deficiency can impair human health severely and cause iodine deficiency disorders (IDD), including endemic goiter, endemic cretinism, endemic subclinical cretinism, and so on. From 2838 to 2698 B. C. , China had made effort to control endemic goiter. However, the large-scale prevention work had not started in a real sense until the founding of the New China. At that time, all regions of China except Shanghai were affected by endemic goiter at different levels. Supply of iodized salt, iodized oil, and iodine-rich foods, iodization of drinking water and iodinated food were the mainly recommended measures for controlling IDD. The surveillance and assessment systems for IDD elimination in China were well organized and carefully designed. Today, China has eliminated IDD on a national basis in many provinces. It is considered one of the most successful IDD elimination programs in the world and has set an excellent example for the rest of the world. According to the most recent national IDD surveillance survey carried out in 2014, China is in the status of sustainable IDD elimination nation-wide, which is attributed to the leading roles of government, high-quality and sufficient iodized salt supply, comprehensive legislation, regulations, standards and technical proposals, intensive surveillance and assessment, health-related promotional and educational activities, and international collaboration.

2. 1　The Main Manifestations and Harms of Iodine Deficiency

2. 1. 1　What is the Disease Spectrum of Iodine Deficiency on the Human Body?

Iodine Deficiency Disorders（IDD）is the collective name of a series of physiological changes and ill conditions caused by iodine deficiency of the human body. Its main manifestations and harms are shown below:

(1) Iodine deficiency can cause endemic goiter（hereafter refer as goiter）, commonly known as "Thicken Neck".

(2) Severe iodine deficiency in fetal period and infancy period can lead to endemic cretinism（cretinism）, and cretinism patients are characterized with mental retardation, short stature, deaf-mutism, paralysis and special facial features.

(3) Severe iodine deficiency in fetal period and infancy period can also cause the so-called endemic sub-clinical cretinism（or sub-clinical cretinism）, and sub-clinical cretinism patients also suffer from mental retardation or delayed development, in spite of the absence of typical symptoms of cretinism.

(4) Iodine malnutrition in fetal period and infancy period, even mild or moderate iodine deficiency can also affect intelligence quotient.

(5) Prenatal maternal iodine deficiency can result in premature delivery, abortion, stillbirth, congenital malformation and congenital deaf-mutism.

IDD impairs human health seriously in various aspects, and has a very harmful effect on the society, especially on the population quality and economic development.

2. 1. 2　Endemic Goiter

2. 1. 2. 1　How does the Endemic Goiter Appear?

Endemic goiter is an endemic disease caused by regional environmental iodine deficiency and is a specific manifestation of IDD（see Fig. 2.1, left）. It is a consequence of compensatory reaction to pathological lesion occurred to thyroid tissue in the case of lack of iodine intake. Its main character and symptom is thyroid enlargement. If the human body is lack of iodine intake, a large number of small follicles will proliferate in the thyroid tissue, each of follicle cavities becomes small and stores less colloid, while the total thyroid volume is enlarged. When the demand of the human body for hormone levels is satisfied, the thyroid follicles remain in a state of "restoration", that is, the follicles swell up, the follicle cavities are full of colloid and the epithelial cells are in the shape of cube. If the environment is sustained deficient in iodine and therefore the human body is standing lack of iodine, the above proliferation and restoration will be intensified and prolonged, increasingly, resulting in diffuse goiter. Severe and long-term iodine deficiency tends to cause intensive proliferation and restoration of thyroid tissue, but it changes a swollen thyroid unevenly. Some parts show obviously excessive proliferation due to their sensitivity to thyroid stimulating hormone (TSH) while other parts show obviously excessive restoration, frequently, the unbalance forms one or more nodules in the diffuse and swollen gland at the early stage. When the enlarged nodule is surrounded by the hyperplasic fibrous tissue, it turns from diffuse goiter into nodular goiter, and some nodules undergo secondary changes such as degeneration, bleeding and necrosis. The degenerated tissue can cause cystic degeneration or form cyst after experiencing liquidation and bleeding. The hyperplasic fibrous tissue can form scar calcinosis, calcification and even ossification, and new nodules may occur in the fibrous tissue or follicle cavities wall. Ultimately, the entire thyroid gland will be replaced by old and new nodules with different sizes. In the early stage of diffuse goiter, the lesion is reversible and can recover through appropriate iodine supplementation measures, but will develop into irreversible nodular goiter in the case of nodular formation due to repeated and excessive proliferation and restoration.

2.1.2.2 What are the Clinical Manifestations of Endemic Goiter?

Mostly, endemic goiter is featured by slow onset, and generally, without obvious symptoms except the thickening neck (thyroid enlargement). It is generally found during physical examination or professional survey; however, when the thyroid is enlarged to a certain extent, it can give rise to obvious clinical symptoms, such as thicken neck, dyspnea (difficult breathing), dysphasia (swallowing difficulty) and hoarseness. During the process of prevention, control and surveillance of IDD, the goiter is examined by palpation and is categorized by its size into three degrees: 0, I and II; furthermore, it is classified into three types: diffuse, nodular and mixed

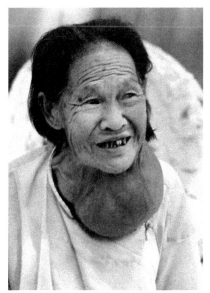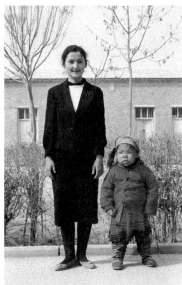

Fig. 2. 1 Endemic goiter and endemic cretinism patients. Left: An endemic goiter woman. Right: a health girl and an endemic cretinism woman.(from China Health Pictorial)

goiter. The laboratory examination indexes, such as thyroid function of patients with endemic goiter are normal and have no significantly difference with those of local residents without goiter. All patients with goiter are characterized with low urinary iodine level and elevated thyroglobulin (Tg) level.

2. 1. 2. 3   How to Diagnose the Endemic Goiter?

According to Chinese latest diagnostic criteria for endemic goiter (WS 276-2007), the following requirements must be satisfied to diagnose a person with endemic goiter：

(1) The person must reside in an iodine-deficient area.

(2) Palpation or B-ultrasonic examination reveals thyroid enlargement or non-enlarged thyroid with nodule.

(3) Hyperthyroidism, thyroiditis and thyroid tumor have been excluded.

If the goiter rate of children aged 8-10 years in an iodine-deficient area is greater than 5% and their median urinary iodine is less than $100\mu g/L$, then the endemic goiter prevails in this area and it should be cautioned as a public health problem. The goiter rate is the percentage of patients with goiter (the sum of patients with goiter at degree Ⅰ and degree Ⅱ by palpation, or patients with goiter by B-ultrasonic examination) to the total number of persons that have undergone the test. When goiter rates resulting from palpation and B-ultrasonic examination are different, results of the B-ultrasonic examination shall be prioritized.

2.1.3　Endemic Cretinism

2.1.3.1　How does the Endemic Cretinism Appear?

Endemic cretinism is an endemic disease mainly characterized with developmental brain disorders and delayed physical development (see Fig. 2.1, right). It is caused by local environmental iodine deficiency and is one of clinical manifestations of iodine deficiency which poses the most severe threat to the human being. Its main clinical manifestations are relatively severe mental retardation, deaf-mutism, motor nerve dysfunction and delayed physical development, the so-called dullness, pygmyism, deafness, dumbness and paralysis. The disease is mainly developmental brain disorders and delayed physical development as a result of insufficient thyroid hormones due to iodine deficiency in the critical period for brain development (the embryonic period and the early postnatal period) and the growth period.

In the case of iodine deficiency in the critical period for brain development (three months after pregnancy to two years after birth), the brain will be impaired firstly due to lack of thyroid hormones. An increase of T_3 has an obvious compensatory effect on other tissues rather than the brain tissue. Moreover, little of T_4 enters brain cells due to a reduction of the T_4, afterwards, resulting in the reduction of T_3, which is transformed from T_4 through deiodination in brain cells. Therefore, thyroid hypofunction (hereafter referred as hypothyroidism) during this period may severely affect proliferation, differentiation and migration of brain cells as well as axon growth and synapse formation, thereby leading to mental retardation, movement disorders and deafness. If the problem of iodine deficiency sustained even after birth, or due to atrophy of thyroid gland, the persistent hypothyroidism will affect the protein synthesis and therefore cause a series of issues such as short stature, retardation of bone age, delayed development of sexual organs, abnormality of cartilage, muscle, hair and finger nail, and so on.

2.1.3.2   What are Clinical Manifestations of Endemic Cretinism?

According to clinical manifestations, endemic cretinism is categorized into three types as below：

Neurologic Cretinism. It is the most common subtype, globally distributed in most countries, including China. Clinically, main manifestations include obvious mental retardation and nerve injury syndrome（hearing ability, speech and motor nerve dysfunctions）. Its main features are as follows：（1）Obvious mental retardation；（2）Deaf-mutism；（3）Motor nerve dysfunction, which is manifested by spastic paralysis, gesture and gait disturbances at varying degrees；（4）Mild physical underdevelopment with a nearly normal stature；（5）Goiter, inconspicuous hypothyroidism.

Myxedematous Cretinism. It has only been found in some countries and regions in South Asia, Africa（Zaire and Congo）, and northwest provinces of China（Xinjiang, Qinghai, Gansu, Ningxia and Inner Mongolia）. Its main clinical manifestations show hypothyroidism characterized with myxedema, which are：（1）Myxedema；（2）Short stature or dwarf；（3）Delayed sexual maturation；（4）Facial features of cretinism；（5）Mental retardation, but it is slighter than that of neurologic cretinism.

Mixed（with Features of Both Neurologic Cretinism and Myxedematous Cretinism）. It prevails in the area with both myxedematous cretinism and neurologic cretinism. Its main features are shown below：（1）Obvious nerve injury；（2）Overt hypothyroidism；（3）Some cases have more features of neurologic cretinism；（4）Some cases have more features of myxedematous cretinism.

According to the illness condition of patient, endemic cretinism is graded into "mild", "moderate" and "severe", mainly based on the six aspects of patient capability（see Table 2.1）.

2.1.3.3   How to Diagnose the Endemic Cretinism

Essential Conditions for Diagnosis of Endemic Cretinism：（1）From epidemiology aspect, the patient was born and lived in an IDD endemic area；（2）Clinical manifestations show mental retardation or hypophrenia in different degrees, and the intelligence quotient（IQ）less than or equal to 54.

Supplementary Conditions for Diagnosis of Endemic Cretinism：（1）Nervous system disorder：mainly including motor nerve disorder, hearing disorder and speech

Table 2.1　Summary Sheet of Clinical Grading of Endemic Cretinism

	Mild	Moderate	Severe
（ⅰ）Living ability	Can look after himself/herself in daily life	Can basically look after himself/herself in daily life	Can barely look after himself/herself in daily life
（ⅱ）Labor capacity	Capable of doing general housework and labor, but hardly to learn complex housework and labor	Capable of doing simple housework and labor	Incapable of doing labor
（ⅲ）Verbal comprehension	Can basically understand simple words	Can only understand single phrase or simple words	Unable to understand the language
（ⅳ）Arithmetic capability	Difficult in doing arithmetic operations	Can do simple addition and subtraction or plus-minus operation of material objects	Has no concept of number
（ⅴ）Language competence	Can speak simple sentences, but cannot speak clearly	Can speak several simple words	Absolute mute, or can only speak simple or utter single word
（ⅵ）Hearing ability	Can hear speech with normal loudness；can hear murmur from one meter behind.	Can hear speech with normal loudness from one meter behind	Stone deaf, or responsive to loud shout from one meter behind.

disorder；(2) Thyroid dysfunctions：mainly including delayed physical development, facial features of cretinism, clinical hypothyroidism and abnormal hormone level.

2. 1. 4　Endemic Sub-Clinical Cretinism

2. 1. 4. 1　How to Distinguish Endemic Sub-Clinical Cretinism from Endemic Cretinism?
Endemic sub-clinical cretinism is a very mild cretinism caused by regional environmental iodine deficiency. It features with slightly mental retardation；the pathogenesis of endemic sub-clinical cretinism is the same as that of endemic cretinism, and mild impairment caused by iodine deficiency is the basic reason for the disease. Patients with endemic sub-clinical cretinism do not present typical manifestations of endemic cretinism, but have some common clinical symptoms. According to a survey, the prevalence of endemic sub-clinical cretinism in iodine-

deficient areas is much higher than that of endemic cretinism, which significantly affect the quality of population in endemic areas, and thereby causing a serious issue in public health.

2. 1. 4. 2   What are the Clinical Manifestations of the Sub-Clinical Cretinism?

Main Clinical Manifestations: (1) Mild mental retardation: the IQ ranges between 55 and 69, namely the so-called weak intelligence, which is the prominent feature of endemic sub-clinical cretinism; (2) Mild nerve injury: It can only be found by adopting an elaborate examination method: 1) Psychomotor dysfunction: prolonged response time, easy fatigability and absence accuracy of action. 2) Mild hearing disorder: patients are usually not deaf, but the following results such as increased threshold values of hearing ability, abnormal high frequency or low frequency can be found at the time of examination. Also, mild increased tendon reflex, increase of EEG (Electroencephalogram) slow waves as well as positive reactions including AEP (Auditory evoked potentials) may be found; (3) Mild thyroid dysfunctions: the indexes can restore completely to normal levels after iodine supplementation. In addition, the height, weight and head circumference of some patients with endemic sub-clinical cretinism are inferior to average values due to lack of thyroid hormones. Retardation of bone age or poor closure of epiphyses tends to be a sensitive index for endemic sub-clinical cretinism.

2.2   The Story of IDD Discovery

IDD is an ancient disease of human being. One of the oldest descriptions about goiter is from the legendary Chinese emperor Shen Nong (2838-2698 B.C.), who, in his book "Shen Nong's Herbal" mentioned the seaweed as an efficacious remedy against goiter. At the beginning of the 7th century B.C., the "Classic of Mountains and Seas (Shan Hai Jing)", an ancient book of China, also recorded endemic goiter and attributed its occurrence to a poor water quality. "Spring and Autumn Annals" by Lv Buwei in the year 239 described that "there are many bald persons and patients with goiter in paticular area", which indicated that the author was aware of a relationship between environmental factors and endemic goiter. During a period of 454-473, "Excerpts of Prescriptions" based on the etiology, firstly categorized goiter into two classes which were similar to today's cystic goiter and nodular goiter. In terms of goiter treatment, a total of 26 prescriptions were formed contain seaweed, kelp, or their combination with other ingredients, of which one prescription included only deer's thyroid. The one-ingredient prescription contained merely deer thyroid was initially collected in "Seng Shi Fang", a book written in "the Northern and Southern Dynasties of China" (420-589). Afterwards, China continued to use animal thyroid to treat the disease. "The General Treatise on the Cause and Symptoms of Diseases" authored by Chao Yuanfang in Sui Dynasty (610) explicitly described the relationship between "goiter" and water and soil. According to "the Supplement to Valuable Prescriptions" authored by Sun Simiao, a famous doctor in Tang Dynasty (682), nearly all prescriptions against goiter involved marine products such as seaweeds, kelp and sea clam, etc. and some prescriptions also utilized deer thyroid to treat endemic goiter. Between 1127 and 1279, a book named as "Confucians' Duties to Their Parents-Goiter" written in Jin Dynasty stated that "brown seaweed, marine algae and kelp are all marine products, and they can be used to treat the goiter by putting them in a water jar and eating them constantly", proposing a method for prevention and control of the goiter. Li Shizhen, another famous medical expert, (Ming Dynasty, 1552-1578) introduced preparations of pig and deer thyroids in his "Compendium of Materia Medica", a medical masterpiece. Therefore, China has a long history of centuries for knowing of goiter and using seaweeds and animal thyroid to treat the disease.

In 1930s, an American scholar and a Japanese military surgeon wrote epidemiologic reports on endemic goiter prevalence in Zunhua of Hebei Province and Chengde of Rehe Province. As for Chinese scholars' epidemiologic reports on endemic goiter, we should firstly mention the survey report on the 37 counties of Yunnan Province made by Yao Xunyuan and Yao Yongzheng between 1940 and 1942. Because of this report, salt iodization was carried out in the Yipinglang salt mine of Yunnan Province in the middle of 1940s, marking the start of the large-scale prevention and control of IDD in China. In the second year after the founding of the New China (1946), Yang Xiufeng, the Governor of Hebei Province, led a delegation to Qianxi County, a time-honored revolutionary base in Hebei Province, and found that the county was prevailed with endemic goiter and dullness. He chose two patients with endemic cretinism and sent them to the Department of Internal Medicine of Tianjin Municipal General Hospital for observation. Unfortunately, no correct diagnosis was made at that time. Under his initiative, a team for goiter prevention and control was established within the Department of Health of Hebei Province at the beginning of 1950s. The team was Chinese first group for prevention and control of endemic goiter. In 1956, Hebei Health Department, Hebei Medical College and Hebei goiter prevention and control team went to Qianxi and Qian' an counties to carry out systematic surveys on endemic goiter, marking the start of integration between prevention and control of endemic goiter and medical colleges in China. However, there was no correct understanding of endemic cretinism in the survey. In 1958, endemic cretinism was reported in Henan and Anhui. In 1959, Tianjin Medical College, under the leadership of Professor Xianyi Zhu, took part in survey for prevention and control of endemic goiter in Hebei. The survey result showed that there were severe problems of endemic cretinism in Tangshan and Chengde of Hebei Province. In 1961, Xianyi Zhu and others organized clinical observations for prevention and control of IDD in the suburbs of Chengde City of Hebei Province. The observation lasted for five years until the beginning of the Great Cultural Revolution. Results of the observation proved that it was iodine deficiency that led to dullness, deaf-mutism and paralysis in mountainous areas in China, which was preventable through measures of iodine supplementation. In 1964 and 1965, Tianjin Medical College and Hebei Provincial Health Department held two academic conferences to present reports on the observation, and to promote the prevention and control of IDD in other areas of China to a certain extent. In 1966, the work was temporarily suspended. In 1960s and 1970s, Jiamusi Medical College systematically reported the endemic goiter and endemic cretinism in Jixian Village, Huachuan County, Jiamusi City, Heilongjiang Province.

As mentioned above, the prevention of IDD was merely experimental before the founding of the New China and benefited only few people. The large-scale prevention work had not started in a real sense until the founding of the New China. Since 1954, manual salt iodization has launched in some endemic areas in Hebei and other provinces in China.

Since 1956, China has gradually expanded the operations of manual iodization to mechanical iodization. By 1958, iodized salt had been popularized in the endemic areas in 18 provinces of China. Since China State Council held the "National Advocacy Meeting for IDD Elimination by the Year 2000" in 1993, China has strived to eliminate IDD. Fig. 2. 2 shows the IDD investigation in Xinjiang in 2007. In 1994, China adopted the Universal Salt Iodization and mainly attained the goal of Universal Salt Iodization in 1996. In 2000, China had basically achieved the stage goal of eliminating IDD. According to the evaluation report made by China national assessment team in 2007, China had attained its goal of IDD elimination. From 2007 to now, China has been in the state of sustained elimination of IDD.

2. 3   Distribution of IDD?

2. 3. 1   Which Regions are Affected by IDD?

IDD is prevalent at different levels in most countries in the world due to the global iodine deficiency distribution. Before the appearance of human beings, the mellow soil layer of the earth was rich in iodine. After the earth entered the quaternary ice age 180,000 years ago, most of its lands were covered by ice layers; later on, the ice layers thawed and the mellow soils on the surface of the earth were washed out to sea. But the soils that regenerated afterwards contain extremely small amount of iodine, accounting for merely one tenth of that of the original soils, causing the global iodine deficiency. In some mountainous areas, semi-mountainous areas, hills, river valleys and fluvial regions, iodine deficiency is even worse, indicating that the occurrence and prevalence of IDD are closely related to the physic-geographical environments of endemic area.

The main epidemiological feature of IDD is distinct regional distribution. IDD exists in all countries except Iceland, a country boosts flourishing fishery and high consumption of sea fishes containing iodine. In the world, the Himalaya Mountains, Papua New Guinea and the Congo River Basin are most severely influenced by IDD. The Andes Mountains in Latin America, the Great Lakes Basin in North America, the Alps and the Pyrenees Mountains are also hit seriously by the disease. In Asia, the

Indian Kashmir and the vast areas on the both sides of the Himalaya Mountains are the most severe iodine-deficient areas in the world. Globally, IDD dominantly spread in the three less-developed continents of Asia, Africa and Latin America.

China is one of the countries with wide distribution of IDD. All of the 31 provinces, municipalities, autonomous regions and the Xinjiang Production and Construction Corps except Shanghai suffer from the prevalence of endemic goiter in different degrees. Geographically, main IDD endemic areas of China are listed below：

Northeast China：Sanjiang Plain, Greater Khingan Mountains and Lesser Khingan Mountains in Heilongjiang, Changbai Mountains in Jilin；North China：Yanshan Mountain in Hebei, the mountainous area in the south of Inner Mongolia, Taihang Mountain at the border of Hebei and Shanxi, Lvliang Mountains in Shanxi, Yimeng Mountains in Shandong；Northwest China：Qinling Mountains in Shaanxi, Longnan Mountains in Gansu, Liupanshan in Ningxia, the agricultural region in the north east Qinghai, the agricultural regions around the Tarim Basin in Xinjiang, some regions at the northern foot of Tianshan Mountain；Southwest China Daba Mountain in the north east of Sichuan and Daliang Mountains and Xiaoliang Mountains in the south west of the province, Dehong Prefecture in the west Yunnan, the mountainous areas in the east, southeast and southwest of Guizhou, Tibet and the Yarlungzangbo River Valley at the northern foot of the Himalaya Mountains；Central South China：the mountainous areas in the west and northwest of Guangxi, north of Guangdong and west of Hunan, as well as the Dabie Mountains and Xianxialing Mountains in Hubei and the Wuyi Mountains in Fujian.

The overall rule of geographic distribution of IDD：The order of the number of patients with IDD（from the highest to the lowest）：mountainous areas, hills, plains, coastal areas；inland areas；the upper reaches of inland rivers, the lower reaches of the inland rivers；agricultural areas, pastoral areas. Fig.2.2 and Fig.2.3 showed the natural scene of IDD endemic area in Guizhou and Xinjiang, respectively.

2.3.2　What is the Time Distribution of IDD?

In the early years after the liberation of China, there were 20 million patients with endemic goiter. Between 1959 and 1977, amongst the over 26 million persons in 28

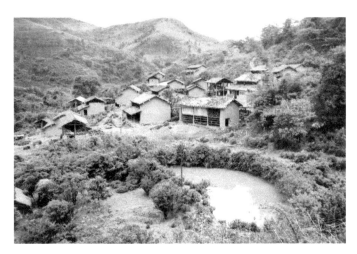

Fig. 2. 2　Natural scenary of IDD endemias in Guizhou（from China Health Pictorial）.

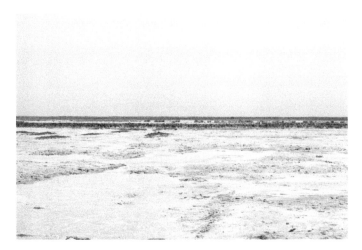

Fig. 2. 3　Natural scenary of IDD endemias in Hetian region of Xinjiang.（This area is far from sea and severe iodine deficiency. Local residents get local salt very conveniently because of rich local salt resources. However, the local salt does not contain iodine, and the long-term consumption of this local salt lead to the cretinism prevalence.）

provinces, municipalities and autonomous regions, the prevalence rate of endemic goiter was 8. 3% ; according to a summary involving 26 provinces, municipalities and autonomous regions, made by Yu Zhiheng in 1983, China prevalence rate of endemic goiter was 12. 85% and that of endemic cretinism was 0. 66%. After comprehensive prevention & control measures including salt iodization and administration of iodized oil in endemic area, the disease had been put under control in other regions except Xinjiang and Tibet. In 1994, when the Universal Salt Iodization had not yet been adopted, there were 1,807 endemic counties according to the former criteria, with 7.99 million patients with endemic goiter and 187,000 patients with typical endemic cretinism. In 1995, the goiter rate of children aged 8-10 years in China was 20.4%. After the adoption of Universal Salt Iodization, the goiter rate of children aged 8-10 in China was 5.0% (by palpation) in 2005, up to the national standard, but that of 5 provinces were higher than 10% and of 12 provinces ranged between 5% and 10%. China conducted IDD surveillance activities in 2011 and 2014 respectively. Data showed that the goiter rates of children aged 8-10 years were 2.4% and 2.6% resepectively, indicating that China has been in the state of sustained IDD elimination at the national level. According to the results of the two surveillance survey, only the goiter rates of Chongqing and Shandong were higher than 5%, while that of other provinces, municipalities, autonomous regions and Xinjiang Production and Construction Corps were lower than 5%.

2.3.3　Which Group of Populations Is More Susceptible to IDD?

Age: IDD may occur to people at any age, and causes the greatest damages to infants aged 0-2 years, children, pregnant women and lactating women. In IDD endemic areas, endemic goiter usually occurs to adolescents and its prevalence rate rises with age and declines after the middle age. More severe the endemic condition of an area is, earlier the goiter onset age of inhabitants in the area is. The occurrence of endemic cretinism is caused by severe iodine deficiency in fetal period and neonatal period. Therefore, iodine supplementation is particularly important for pregnant women, lactating women and infants aged 0-2 years.

　　Gender: The prevalence of endemic goiter among children under 10 years old does not differ significantly by gender; however, the prevalence of goiter among female adolescents is higher than that among male adolescents. The more severe the endemic condition of the area is, the smaller the difference of prevalences between male and female is.

　　Village-Based and Family-Related Occurrence: Endemic cretinism only occurs in the areas with severe iodine deficiency, but not in all severe iodine-deficient areas. Moreover, patients with endemic cretinism are not evenly distributed, but tend to cluster in one or more natural villages, thus causing "villages of fool", and endemic cretinism is also markedly related to family.

2.4   Classifications of IDD Endemic Areas in China

2.4.1   What is the Definition of the IDD Endemic Areas?

According to the stipulation of Delimitation for the Endemic Areas of Iodine Deficiency Disorders（GB16005-2009）, an area on the basis of township can be considered as an IDD endemic area if it complies with all indexes as follows: (1) Water iodine: the median of iodide content in drinking water is less than $10\mu g/$ L; (2) Urinary iodine: the median urinary iodine of children aged 8-10 is less than $100\mu g/L$, and the number of samples with the concentration less than $50\mu g/L$ accounts for over 20% of the total number; (3) Goiter rate: the goiter rate of children aged 8-10 is greater than 5%.

2.4.2   How to Distinguish the Different Classification of IDD Endemic Areas?

According to Delimitation for the Endemic Areas of Iodine Deficiency Disorders （GB16005-2009）, China IDD endemic areas are classified into mild, moderate and severe endemic areas as follows:

Mild IDD Endemic Area: the urinary iodine of children aged 8-10 is greater than or equal to $50\mu g/L$ and less than $100\mu g/L$; the number of samples with the concentration less than $50\mu g/L$ accounts for 20% or above of the total number; the goiter rate of children aged 8-10 ranges between 5% and 20%, without the occurrence of endemic cretinism.

Moderate IDD Endemic Area: the urinary iodine of children aged 8-10 is greater than or equal to $20\mu g/L$ and less than $50\mu g/L$; the goiter rate of children aged 8-10 ranges between 20% and 30%; with or without the occurrence of endemic cretinism.

Severe IDD Endemic Area: the urinary iodine of children aged 8-10 is less than 20μg/L; the goiter rate of children aged 8-10 is greater than or equal to 30%; with the occurrence of endemic cretinism.

If the above three indexes disagree with each other, the goiter rate of children aged 8-10 shall be prioritized.

2.5　Prevention Strategies and Measures of IDD?

2.5.1　How about the Effect of Iodized Salt on IDD?

As the recommended strategy for controlling IDD, the Universal Salt Iodization requires that all edible salt, including salt for food processing and household use, is iodized. Today, 76% of the households worldwide use iodized salt and, as a result, the number of iodine-deficient countries has decreased from 110 in 1993 to 30 in 2014. In China, the IDD prevention and control efforts had started since 1940s. From 1940 to 1942, Yao Yongzheng and Yao Xunyuan from the Kunming Health Bureau, surveyed goiter patients in 37 counties of Yunnan province and carried out salt iodization at Yipinglang Salt Mine of the province based on the survey. Since 1950s, manual salt iodization had initiated in some endemic areas in Hebei and Shaanxi provinces of China. In the 1960s, machines began to be used for mixing the iodine into salt. Since 1965, China has gradually expanded the operation of mechanical iodization. In 1985, iodized salt had been popularized in 18 provinces. In August 1994, the Chinese former Premier Li Peng signed the No.163 Decree of the State Council to issue the Management Regulations on Elimination of Iodine Deficiency Hazards by Salt Iodization. In 1995, the State Council launched a program for salt iodization, with a total investment of RMB 980 million including a US $ 27 million loan from the World Bank for upgrading technologies and equipment of 108 designated iodized salt production enterprises. In 2002, iodized salt was produced by the salt industry company（Fig 2.4）, China production capacity of iodized salt reached 8.18 million tons, which could meet the consumption demand of the whole country. The National Development and Reform Commission, the Ministry of Industry and Information Technology and corresponding local governments have effectively strengthened the management of production and marketing of edible salt, ensured sufficient supply of iodized salt, and established a broad sale network. China State Administration for Industry and Commerce, supported by salt-related authorities, has taken a series of actions to crack down the illegal sales of non-iodized salt, unqualified and fake iodized salt so as to maintain the normal order of the salt market.

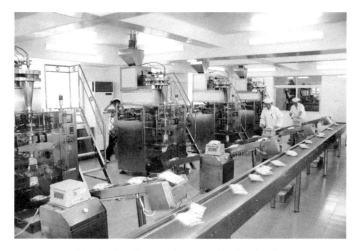

Fig. 2. 4　The production of iodized salt.

2. 5. 2　How to Adjust and Control the Iodized Salt Concentration

In 1979, China State Council endorsed the Interim Procedures of Salt Iodization for Prevention and Control of Endemic Goiter drafted by the Ministry of Health, the Ministry of Light Industry, the Ministry of Commerce, the Ministry of Food and All China Federation of Supply and Marketing Cooperatives. The Procedures proposed that the ideal proportional range of salt iodization should be 1/50000-1/20000. In 1993, the State Council held the "National Advocacy Meeting for IDD Elimination by the Year 2000", according to the requirements on prevention and control work as well as the regulations including the Outline of China for IDD Elimination by the Year 2000 and the Criteria for Elimination of IDD（GB16006-1995）, the iodine concentration of iodized salt（calculated based on the number of iodide ions）shall meet the requirements below: 50mg/kg for production, no less than 40mg/kg for transportation, no less than 30mg/kg for marketing and no less than 20mg/kg for household. In consideration of the excessive concentration of iodized salt during transportation due to the absence of upper limit of iodization level in the stipulations on salt iodine concentration that was specified in 1993, China adjusted its iodization level in 1997 based on the IDD surveillance result, namely, stipulating that the salt iodine concentration must not be greater than 60mg/kg. In October 2000, the Ministry of Health announced to reduce the iodization level of iodized salt from 50mg/kg to 35 ± 15mg/kg, and revised the corresponding national standards, for example, the Edible Salt (GB5461-2000) specified that the iodine concentration (calculated based on the number of iodide ions) shall be in the range of 35 ± 15mg/kg. As mentioned above, the Ministry of Health readjusted the iodized salt concentration in March 2012, reducing the average iodine concentration of edible salt (calculated based on the number of iodide ions) to 20-30mg/kg. Each province can choose one or two values of iodized salt concentration corresponding to its actual situation (Fig. 2.5).

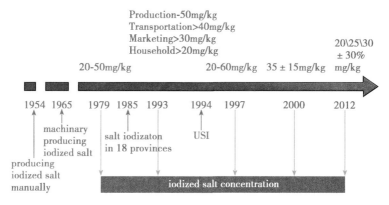

Fig. 2.5　China adjustments of iodized salt concentration.

2.5.3　How about the Effect of Iodized Oil on IDD?

2.5.3.1　*Type, Dosage Form and Iodine Content of Iodized Oil*

Iodized oil is a type of organic iodide that is produced by additive reaction between vegetable oil and hydrogen iodide (HI), and its scientific name is ethyl iodized oil. Clinically, there are three types of iodized oil for prevention and control of endemic goiter and endemic cretinism, namely iodinated linoleic rapeseed oil, iodinated walnut oil and iodinated soya oil. Besides injection, iodized oil also has dosage forms of soft capsule and micro-capsule granule for oral administration, the former contains 0.2g iodine per capsule and the latter contains 0.2g iodine per packet. Micro-capsule granule is a type of new dosage form, which is made of natural and synthetic high polymer material (Arabic gum is generally used) containing liquid, with a diameter of 1-5000. It has advantages of delayed release in stomach, higher stability, absence of bitter taste which is suitable for oral administration and changed administration route, etc. In addition, it is convenient for storage and transportation and is suitable for children.

2.5.3.2 Administration Route and Dosage of Iodized Oil

As a supplement to iodized salt, iodized oil is suitable for remote and geographically-inaccessible areas, the vast areas with a sparse population, in those areas the residents cannot commercially get access to edible salt but produce salt by their own, as well as those areas without supply or effective supply of iodized salt, especially for those areas with high prevalence of endemic cretinism and underdeveloped economy. Particularly, women of childbearing age in some areas with high prevalence of endemic cretinism shall also be injected with or taken iodized oil, even if iodized salt has been supplied in such areas, to prevent the occurrence of endemic cretinism(Fig. 2.6).

(1) Intramuscular injection site: hip for children and deltoid for adults. The injection must be made slowly at an accurate site. When it has been decided to inject iodized oil for the inhabitants in a certain area, the injection shall be completed as soon as possible. Generally, all persons aged 0-45 in the endemic area shall be injected with iodized oil, except for those who have large nodular goiter and severe liver and kidney diseases, etc.

(2) The appropriate dosage for oral administration of iodized oil is generally 1.4 times of that intramuscular injection. If an adult shall receive an intramuscular injection of 500mg iodized oil, equivalently, he/she shall take orally soft capsules of iodized oil with a dosage of about 700mg, or take orally micro-capsule granules with a dosage that is only approximately same with that of intramuscular injection.

2.5.3.3 Precaution of Oral Administration of Iodized Oil

(1) Strengthening the capacity of community-level prevention and control personnel

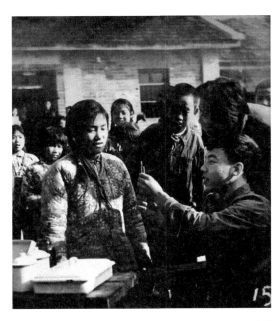

Fig. 2. 6   Iodized oil was taken in Hubei. (from Hubei Province
Center for Disease Control and Prevention)

so as to enable them to master techniques for prevention and processing of
indications, side effects and accidents; (2) Completing intensive organization and
publicity work of iodized oil administration, so as to obtain support from inhabitants
and reduce the "mass adverse reaction"; (3) Iodized oil must be taken under the
guidance and supervision of medical staff; (4) Iodized oil must be taken after a meal,
and must not be taken in an empty stomach; (5) Iodized oil is forbidden for patients
with cold, fever and gastroenteritis; (6) Iodized oil is forbidden for patients with
severe heart, liver, lung and kidney diseases, used with caution for patients with a
history of medicine allergy, and is forbidden for patients (including their immediate
family members) with iodine allergy; (7) Forbidden in principle for patients with
nodular goiter, hyperthyroidism and other diseases that is not allowed with an
administration of iodized oil.

2. 5. 4   Is there Any Other Methods for IDD Prevention and Control?

2. 5. 4. 1   *Iodization of Drinking Water*
Water is essential for daily life and is another ideal approach for iodine

supplementation besides salt, but it is rather difficult to be collected for iodization due to its wide distribution. However, in certain special environments, water iodization is an effective measure for solving the problem of iodine deficiency. The methods for water iodization include: (1) Direct iodization of drinking water; (2) Iodine sustained-release device; (3) Iodine diffuser with iodine-containing silica gel; (4) Iodization of water for crop irrigation. Three types of iodine-related products are used for iodization: potassium iodate (KIO_3), potassium iodide (KI) and iodine (I_2). Iodization of drinking water is virtually the safest iodization method, without negative side-effects. It can be used in the areas where iodized salt is not supplied or promoted. From the perspective of disinfection of drinking water, iodization by I_2 is more effective than potassium iodate (KIO_3) and potassium iodide (KI), but it requires more iodine and thus costs more compared with other methods.

2.5.4.2　*Iodinated Food*

The government of Zepu County of Xinjiang had ever used iodinated bread (20mg/kg) to prevent and control endemic goiter and gained remarkable effect. Also, someone had used iodine-containing edible oil, iodine-containing soybean sauce, and iodine-containing brick tea for prevention and control of endemic goiter.

2.5.4.3　*Supply of Iodine-Rich Foods*

If iodine-deficient areas are systematically supplied with iodine-rich foods including brown seaweed, marine algae, sea fish and sea clam, it will improve the nutrition of residents in endemic areas and raise the effect of prevention and control of IDD.

In IDD endemic areas, if livestock and poultry are fed with iodine-containing fodder, or animals are raised with seaweeds and trash fish meal, the iodine content of egg, milk and meat will increase, and achieve a remarkable effect for growth and reproduction of animals.

2.5.4.4　*Advocacy of Rational Nutrition and Improvement of Dietary Composition*

IDD in nature is a type of nutritional disorder mainly caused by iodine deficiency. Some factors including low protein, low calorie, lack of certain vitamins and inorganic salts as well as inappropriate proportion of nutrients can affect the iodine absorption and utilization of human body, or hinder the synthesis of thyroid hormones. Therefore, nutritional enhancement and dietary improvement cannot eradicate the iodine deficiency, but can lower its incidence rate and significantly improve the health conditions.

2.6　IDD Surveillance

2.6.1　Surveillance and Assessment Systems for IDD Elimination in China

The surveillance and evaluation systems for IDD elimination in China are well organized and carefully designed. The surveillance systems routinely used to monitor salt quality, household consumption of iodized salt and population-based iodine status are collectively named as the Chinese Surveillance System of Iodine Deficiency Disorders（CSSIDD）（top left corner of Fig. 2.7）. In addition, the government evaluates key stages of the work and performs special surveys on specific issues for additional information. Besides the main intervention strategy of the Universal Salt Iodization, China has also taken conventional intervention measures for high-risk populations（including pregnant women and lactating women）as well as supplementary intervention measures such as administration of emergency iodized oil capsules and free distribution of iodized salt in areas with low coverage of iodized salt（bottom right of Fig. 2.7）.

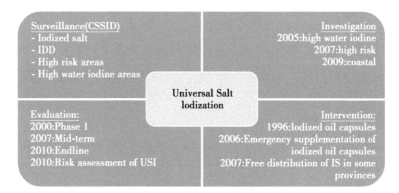

Fig. 2.7　IDD surveillance in China.

2.6.2 When to Launch IDD Surveillance?

China performs national IDD surveillance survey regularly (it was carried out every two years until 2000 when IDD was basically eliminated at a national level and thereafter it was conducted at an interval of 3-6 years) to evaluate goiter prevalence and the iodine nutritional level of the population. The national IDD survey had been made respectively in 1995, 1997, 1999, 2002, 2005 and 2011. The latest national IDD survey was conducted in 2014. The national iodized salt survey was carried out from 1996. It aimed to monitor the coverage rate of iodized salt and consumption rate of qualified iodized salt. Since 2007, an intensified survey named high risk survey had been performed in the low coverage of iodized salt areas and areas with historical cretinism patients, and it was ceased at 2012. China began to monitor non-iodized salt in 2005 through iodized salt survey. It aimed to monitor the coverage of iodized salt, goiter rate, and urinary iodine concentration of children aged 8-10 years. High-risk area surveillance was supplemented to the CSSIDD in 2008. Its purpose is to monitor the prevalence of IDD and the iodine nutritional level of the population in high-risk areas for adjustment of prevention & control measures if necessary.

2.6.3 How to Carry out IDD Surveillance?

The CSSIDD consists of two parts: (1) surveillance on the salt iodine concentration and quality conducted by the salt administration and relevant government departments in the process of production, wholesale and marketing process; (2) surveillance conducted by health authorities over household coverage with iodized salt at county level and population-based iodine status at provincial and national levels. The "National IDD Surveillance process" consists of four parts as shown in Fig. 2. 8.

The implementation plan of national IDD survey as part of the CSSIDD (surveillance over household coverage with iodized salt and population-based iodine status conducted by health authorities) has been revised several times, the early "National IDD Surveillance Plan" being implemented was jointly issued by the former Ministry of Health (MOH), the National Development and Reform Commission (NDRC), the State Administration for Industry and Commerce (SAIC) and the General Administration of Quality Supervision, Inspection and Quarantine

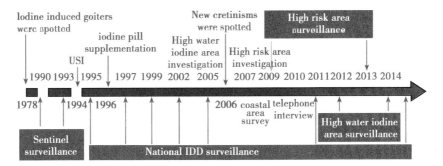

Fig. 2. 8   The national IDD surveillance process.

(GAQSIQ) at the end of 2007. It was revised in 2012 and re-issued by the Center for Endemic Disease Control, Chinese Center for Disease Control and Prevention.

The IDD survey is carried out based on the provincial level. In each province, 30 units are randomly sampled by the method of "population proportion sampling". In each unit, one primary school is randomly sampled, and 50 students aged 8-10 are sampled out of each school for examination of thyroid volume, test of urinary iodine concentration, and collection of salt samples from their households. Since 2011, the assessment of urinary iodine of pregnant women has been included in the sampling frame for IDD surveillance. The Center for Endemic Disease Control, Chinese Center for Disease Control and Prevention is responsible for the management and coordination of China IDD surveillance, while the laboratory quality control is implemented by the National IDD Reference Laboratory.

China national salt surveillance aims to describe the coverage rate of iodized salt at household level and identify high risk areas with lower coverage of iodized salt. It is based on county and conducted once a year in all provinces, municipalities and autonomous regions. Salt iodine concentration is tested by titration in county-level laboratories. Under the supervision of provincial or prefecture-level disease control institution, the survey is carried out by county-level disease control institutions between April 1 and June 5 each year.

In high water iodine areas, the coverage of non-iodized salt is mainly monitored, and the surveillance of goiter and urinary iodine concentration of children aged 8-10 has been started since 2012.

High-risk areas are those areas with iodized salt coverage <80% and have a history of endemic cretinism. IDD surveillance in high-risk areas is based on county so as to rapidly determine the urgent degree of iodine deficiency, which generally implements in the second half of each year. Three townships are randomly selected in each high-risk county and the assessment on suspected endemic cretinism cases, urinary iodine and goiter rate of school children aged 8-10 will be examined. Outpatient and hospital records of county-level hospitals and village health centers are reviewed for locating suspected endemic cretinism cases. Forty children are sampled out of two primary schools per township. In two villages per township, historical or new cases of cretinism are assessed, salt samples are tested from 20 households using semi-quantitative method, and urine samples are collected from 10 women of childbearing age（pregnant women after 2012）. If the assessment results suggest it is necessary for extra iodine supplement, iodized oil capsules are supplied to high-risk populations（pregnant women and lactating women）and iodized salt is supplied locally under the coordination of the health and salt administrations. IDD surveillance in high-risk areas is coordinated and supervised by the Endemic Disease Control Center, Chinese Center for Disease Control and Prevention.

Another part of the CSSIDD is the Laboratory Quality Control Network, which aims to standardize laboratory-operating procedures and test the proficiency of laboratory technicians to guarantee that laboratories at different levels provide scientific and reliable test results. The network is in the charge of the National IDD Reference Laboratory. From January to April each year, before the national iodized salt surveillance starts, the National IDD Reference Laboratory distributes blind samples of urine and salt to the laboratories which takes part in the surveillance and then requests them to provide necessary feedback within a specified time limit. Participating laboratories include all provincial and prefecture-level laboratories for urine and salt tests. If problems occur during laboratory procedures, the National IDD Reference Laboratory will provide a necessary assistance to relevant laboratories for taking corrective measures. Only qualified laboratories can take part in the IDD surveillance.

2.7 Achievements In IDD Prevention and Control of China

2.7.1 Where we stand for IDD Prevention and Control of China

The Chinese government always emphasizes great importance for the prevention and control of IDD. As early as in 1956, China formulated the National Program for Agricultural Development（Draft）, and made explicit stipulations on the prevention and control of endemic goiter. In March 1991, the Chinese government made a solemn commitment to the international community to attain the goal of eliminating IDD in 2000. In August 1993, China's State Council set up a leading group for coordination of IDD elimination headed by State Councilor Peng Peiyun. In 1994, China issued the Management Regulations on Elimination of Iodine Deficiency Damages by Salt Iodization and defined the strategy of implementing the Universal Salt Iodization for prevention and control of IDD.

Since 1995, China had carried out seven large-scale national-level IDD surveillance survey, based on which the standard of salt iodine concentration was adjusted, to supplement iodine in a scientific way and ensure appropriate iodine nutritional level of Chinese inhabitants. In 2000, China announced that it had basically achieved the goal of IDD elimination at national level. At the end of 2010, a total of 28 provinces, municipalities and autonomous regions of China had realized their goals of IDD elimination. Xinjiang, Xizang and Qinghai had attained the goal of basically eliminating IDD. Overall, 97.94% of the counties（cities and districts）in China had attained the goal of IDD elimination. According to the result of China IDD surveillance carried out in 2014, the goiter rate of children（measured by B-ultrasonic method）was 2.6%, below the elimination standard of 5.0%. The coverage rate of iodized salt in China was 96.3%. The consumption rate of qualified iodized salt was 91.5%, which was higher than a clear-cut criterion of 90.0% put forward by the international organization. The median urinary iodine of children was 197.9μg/L, and the iodine nutritional level of the population remained generally in an adequate level（Table 2.2）.

Table 2. 2   Chinese Historical Process of Sustained Elimination of IDD
(technical index)

Index	1995	1997	1999	2002	2005	2011	2014
Iodized salt							
The coverage rate of iodized salt (%)	80. 2	90. 2	93. 9	95. 2	94. 9	98. 0	96. 3
The consumption rate of qualified iodized salt (%)	39. 9	69. 0	80. 6	88. 8	90. 2	95. 3	91. 5
Median of household salt iodine (mg/kg)	16. 2	37. 0	42. 3	31. 4	30. 8	30. 2	24. 8
Urinary iodine							
Proportion of samples with urinary iodine concentration less than 50μg/L	13. 3	3. 5	3. 3	5. 8	5. 6	3. 7	4. 3
Median urinary iodine (μg/L)	164. 8	330. 2	306. 6	241. 2	246. 3	238. 6	197. 9
Disease condition							
Goiter rate (%)	20. 4[*]	9. 6	8. 0	5. 1	4. 0	2. 4	2. 6

Note: [*] indicates the goiter rate was obtained by palpation.

2. 7. 2   Chinese Experience in IDD Prevention and Control

China has accumulated plenty of work experience over the past 20 years since the adoption of Universal Salt Iodization. These experiences include (1) it has established a work mechanism of "government leading, making concerted efforts, emphasizing the importance of prevention, conducting prevention and control in a scientific way, focusing on key points, adjusting measures suitable for local conditions, developing a comprehensive plan and implementing the plan steadily"; (2) it has provided the public with high-quality and sufficient iodized salt, set up and improved sale network that covers both rural and urban areas, and ensured an implementation of the comprehensive prevention and control measures that substantially support salt iodization; (3) it has formulated and revised its laws, regulations, standards and technical proposals, which provide legal, policy and technical supports for the work of IDD elimination; (4) it has intensively carried out surveillance and assessment, to find and resolve issues that occurred during the process of IDD elimination, and further adjust strategies or improve measures for IDD prevention and control；(5) it has extensively engaged in effective health education and promotion activities to broadcast knowledge about IDD prevention and control, to raise the health awareness in the region and to prevent the disease for the general public；(6) it has actively taken part in international cooperation and exchanges to learn experience from other countries and to ensure Chinese IDD elimination stand in an international leading position.

Further Reading

1. Center for Endemic Disease Control, Chinese Center for Disease Control and Prevention.China National Iodine Deficiency Disorders Surveillance Report 2014.

2. SUN DJ. Endemiology. Beijing：People's Medical Publishing House. 2011.

3. Center for Endemic Disease Control, Chinese Center for Disease Control and Prevention. China National Iodine Deficiency Disorders Surveillance Report 1995. Beijing：People's Medical Publishing House, 1999. 3-9.

4. Liu SJ, Su XH, Yu J, et al. Analysis Report of Chinese Iodine Deficiency Disorders in 2002. Chinese Journal of Endemiology. 2003,22(z1)：142-144.

5. Liu P, Su XH, Shen HM, et al. National Iodine Deficiency Disorders：An Analysis of Surveillance Data in 2011. Chinese Journal of Endemiology. 2015,34(3)：181-185.

6. Lv JG, Liu SJ, Sun SQ, et al. China National Iodine Deficiency Disorders Surveillance Report 1997. Beijing：People's Medical Publishing House.2000, 3-21.

7. Ministry of Health of the People's Republic of China. National surveillance program on IDD and high water iodine area surveillance program (on trial), Mar 2012.

8. Ministry of Health of the People's Republic of China.Iodine Concentration in Edible Salt(GB 26878-2011). National Food Safety Standard. People's Medical Publishing House. 2011.

9. The State Technology Supervision Bureau of China. Edible Salt(GB5461-2000). Standards Press of China. 2000.

10. National IDD Surveillance Team. Analysis of Chinese Iodine Deficiency Disorders in 1999. Chinese Journal of Endemiology. 2000, 19(4)：269-271.

11. Su XH, Liu SJ, Shen HM, et al. Analysis Report of Chinese Iodine Deficiency Disorders in 2005. Chinese Journal of Endemiology. 2007, 26(1)：67-69.

12. Ma T, Lu TZ, Yu ZH. Iodine deficiency disorders. Beijing：People's Medical Publishing House.

1993.

13. The north leading group for prevention and control of endemic diseases. The research compilation of preventing and controlling endemic goiter and endemic cretinism. Shenyang: The north leading group for prevention and control of endemic diseases. 1978.

14. The National Standardization Management Committee. Criteria of delimitation for IDD endemic areas（GB16005-1995）. Standards Press of China. 1995.

15. The National Standardization Management Committee. Delimitation for the Endemic Areas of Iodine Deficiency Disorders（GB16005-2009）. Standards Press of China. 2009.

16. Yu ZH. The significant actions for preventing Iodine Deficiency Disorders in home and abroad. Chinese Journal of Preventive Medicine.1994, 6:324-326.

17. Zimmerman M. Global progress against iodine deficiency, new WHO guidelines on iodised salt. Presentation at the Workshop on IDD Prevention and Control Strategies in China, 5-6 November 2014, Beijing.

Chapter 3

Endemic Fluorosis

Zhizhong Guan, **Lihua Wang**, **Dianjun Sun**

Abstract

Endemic fluorosis refers to that individuals living in a region characterized by high levels of fluorine in the drinking water, food and/or air are thereby exposed to excessive amounts of this ion and resulted in general chronic accumulated fluorosis among many of them. In addition to its typical dental and skeletal symptoms, fluorosis extensively damages the whole body, including the brain, liver, kidney, heart, thyroid, etc. The three types of endemic fluorosis resulting from drinking water, coal-burning or drinking-tea types have been identified in China affect 130 million people and for years this situation has been addressed by key national programs for research, prevention and treatment supported by the Chinese government. Through the admirable efforts of scientific researchers and medical professionals, the causes, epidemiology, pathological impairment and pathogenesis of endemic fluorosis are now basically understood. Importantly, the strategy of prevention and control to the disease has been carried out successfully. Thus, endemic fluorosis has been effectively controlled in China and the prevalence of both dental and skeletal fluorosis have been significantly reduced.

3.1 General Introduction to Endemic Fluorosis

3.1.1 Is Fluorine an Essential Trace Element and/or Toxic?

Generally speaking, fluorine is an essential trace element for humans, helping to prevent dental caries (cavities) by converting the hydroxyapatite in tooth enamel into the more resistant fluorapatite.Fluorapatite is not a natural component of human teeth, whereas the main mineral found in natural tooth enamel is hydroxyapatite. Normally, the mineral content of teeth depends on the pH and the concentrations of other substances such as calcium and phosphate in the mouth. In addition to attenuating the breakdown of the teeth by lactic acid-producing bacteria, fluoride enhances and modifies the restoration of the mineral content of teeth in a beneficial manner. In many countries, this ion is added to drinking water (water fluoridation) and toothpaste to prevent dental caries. Other topical fluoride therapies include fluoridated mouth rinses, lozenges, gels, foams and varnishes. It indicates that fluoride therapy may repair rather than prevent damage to the teeth, causing the mineral fluorapatite to be incorporated into damaged tooth enamel.

However, people have very different opinions about water fluoridation, which is not surprising in light of the large number of contradictory findings concerning the benefits and toxicity of systemic fluoride therapy. This debate began roughly 70 years ago, when communities began fluoridating water to prevent tooth decay. After seven decades of studies, every major health organization now agrees that appropriately fluoridated water protects the teeth without posing risks to health.

While almost all water naturally contains some fluoride, the levels in the community water systems that serve most American households have been augmented usually by adding fluoride to reduce tooth decay. Health organizations maintain that this is one of the major reasons fewer people now need the dentures that were so common before widespread fluoridation. Moreover, dental costs are lower and oral health problems have declined in fluoridated communities.

At the same time, anti-water fluoridation activists emphasize that fluoridating water is a form of involuntary medication, causing millions of children to develop dental fluorosis, a discoloration of the teeth that can cause embarrassment and anxiety. In addition, fluoridated water can cause severe bone disease and arthritis, damage the developing brain, impair thyroid function and possibly lead osteosarcoma (bone cancer). Moreover, certain studies have found no consistent or meaningful difference in the prevalence of cavities in fluoridated and non-fluoridated areas.

In view of these considerations and large populations live in regions with endemic fluorosis, we recommend topical application of fluoride to prevent caries, if need, and typically in the form of a fluoride toothpaste or fluoridated mouth rinse.

3. 1. 2   The History and Concept of Endemic Fluorosis

In China and many other developing countries, the negative impact of fluoride, especially in regions of endemic fluorosis, has been considerable. Although the first pathological changes were manifested as skeletal and dental fluorosis, the toxicity by excessive fluoride is now thought to cause extensive impairment of multiple-systems and organs. The countries affected by endemic fluorosis include China, India, Bangladesh, Sri Lanka, Vietnam, Thailand, Iran, Argentina, the USA, Canada, Mexico, Morocco, South Africa, Tanzania, Algeria, Tunis, Egypt, etc. Of these, China and India contain the largest endemic areas where the effects of fluorosis are most severe.

Fluorosis was first recognized at the beginning of the last century, when Greene Vardiman Black, a famous dental researcher and dean of the Northwestern University Dental School of Chicago, USA, observed mottled teeth that Frederick Sumner McKay, a well-known dentist and the president of the Colorado State Dental Association, later showed to be related to drinking water. In 1931, Churchill, the chief chemist at the company headquarters of the Aluminum Company of America in Pennsylvania, reported high concentrations of fluoride in the drinking water in the areas where mottled teeth were prevalent.

Just one year later, the term fluorosis was first used by Moller and Gudjonsson to describe industrial osteosclerosis (skeletal fluorosis). In 1937 Shortt reported 10 cases of fluorosis in India and in the same year Roholm reported 68 cases of industrial fluorosis, in both instances involving system other than the skeleton. In 1976, Waldbott, the chief editor of the international journal, Fluoride, presented research findings concerning non-skeletal fluorosis at an international conference.

In China, endemic fluorosis has a long history. Chinese archeologists have observed dental and skeletal fluorosis in the front teeth and skull fossils of ancient humans living in Xujiayao village in Yanggao County of Shanxi Province, suggesting the possible prevalence of endemic fluorosis about 100,000 years ago. In addition, the "Dingcun people" who inhabited in Xiangfen County of Shanxi Province 100,000 years ago exhibited dental fluorosis in the fossils, and the individuals living under the Xia dynasty 4000 years ago were suffered from skeletal fluorosis. At the time of the Three Kingdoms, Ji Kang living in Kingdom Wei (225-262 A. D.) mentioned 'inhabitants in Shanxi with yellow color teeth' in his writings about maintaining good health, which is considered to be the earliest known description of a connection between mottled teeth and environment.

In 1930, Anderson and colleagues reported 398 cases of dental fluorosis in areas close to Beijing and 109 cases near Taiyuan, China, in the Journal of Dental Research. Furthermore, in *the Lancet* in 1946, the British scholar Lyth described 4 Miao adults with skeletal fluorosis and 134 Miao children with dental fluorosis living in Shimenkan village in the Weining Ethnic Autonomous County of the Guizhou Province, China. During the 1930s to 1960s, Chinese researchers discovered that the fluoride content in drinking water in northeast and northwest China was considerably above the safe level, which was proposed to be related to the elevated prevalence of dental fluorosis in these regions. In 1977, the North China Leading Group of Endemic Disease Prevention and Treatment, under direct control of Central Government, placed endemic fluorosis on the list of Key Diseases to be Prevented and Treated in China.

Today, Chinese scientists have demonstrated clearly that severe endemic fluorosis is found in many provinces and regions of China. In 2010, as many as 1308 endemic areas (counties and cities) had been identified, with a total population of more than 116 million, including 39.5 million patients diagnosed with dental fluorosis and 2.88 million with skeletal fluorosis. The extensive poverty is a direct or indirect cause of the disease, greatly hampering social development. For same time now governments at all levels in China have given great care to the people suffered from the disease in these endemic fluorosis areas and invested considerable effort, equipment and financial resources into investigations, prevention and treatment of endemic fluorosis. Over four decades, Chinese researchers and officials have obtained valuable knowledge concerning the epidemiology, causes, symptoms, pathogenesis, prevention and treatment of endemic fluorosis, much of which has received considerable international acclaim. The systematic project designed to control the sources of fluorine and improve sanitation and health in China has made significant accomplishments, achieving the objectives for prevention and treatment of the disease formulated in the 12ᵗʰ Five-year Program. At present, endemic fluorosis in China is generally under control.

3. 2　Characteristics of Factors that Influence Endemic Fluorosis

The formation of the endemic fluorosis region is related primarily to the accumulation of fluorine in earth shell.

3. 2. 1　How Many Types of Endemic Fluorosis Are There and What Is Their Distribution?

On the basis of route by which fluorine is intaken, the regions of endemic fluorosis fall into three categories.

3. 2. 1. 1　Drinking Water Type of Endemic Fluorosis

The upper limit for fluorine content in drinking water in China is 1. 2 mg/L. The drinking water type of endemic fluorosis is a chronic poisoning caused by drinking water with high level of fluoride (over 1. 2 mg/L) for a long period. The high level of fluoride in water results from the high level of the ion in local rocks and soil.

Surveys performed before 1979 revealed that certain endemic areas, the fluoride content in drinking water was as high as 20.0 mg/L and the prevalences of dental and skeletal fluorosis as high as 100% and 29.8%, respectively, with a great number of patients being handicapped by skeletal fluorosis. During the period of 2005-2008, many of the affected provinces improved their screening of sources of drinking water containing high level of fluorine, using the funding earmarked for public health by the central government. In 2008-2009 a nationwide stratified investigation of endemic fluorosis caused by drinking water was carried out and the geographical distribution and degree of seriousness in various areas clearly identified. By 2014, endemic fluorosis areas caused by drinking water had been shown to be widely scattered across 28 provinces and municipalities, among which Liaoning, Jilin, Heilongjiang, Tianjin, Hebei, Shanxi, Inner Mongolia, Shandong, Henan, Shaanxi, Gansu, Qinghai, Ningxia and Xinjiang are most severely affected. In total, 1055 counties are affected with 61.9 million people at risk, including 18.2 million suffering from dental fluorosis and 1.3 million from skeletal fluorosis (Fig. 3.1).

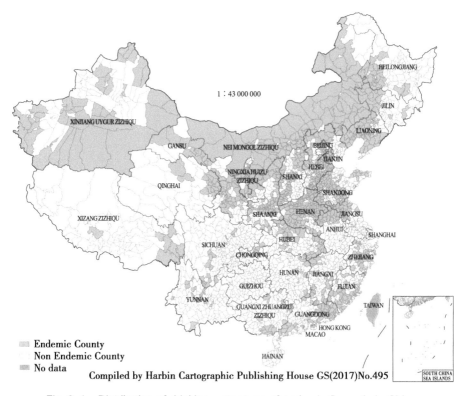

Endemic County
Non Endemic County
No data

Compiled by Harbin Cartographic Publishing House GS(2017)No.495

Fig. 3.1   Distribution of drinking water type of endemic fluorosis in China.

3.2.1.2   Coal-burning Type of Endemic Fluorosis

In 1970s, scientists in Guizhou Province first identified an area in Guizhou, China where endemic fluorosis was not caused by drinking water. The researchers in Guizhou and Hubei provinces confirmed latter that the cause was the burning of coal. The epidemiological survey indicates that the inhabitants in these areas heat, cook and dry grains and vegetables by burning coal containing high level of fluorine in open stoves without chimneys indoors, resulting in food contamination and indoor air pollution with fluorine, which is called coal-burning type of endemic fluorosis. Subsequently, the same type of endemic fluorosis was also found in Yunnan, Sichuan, Hunan, Shaanxi, Chongqing, Jiangxi, Guangxi, Shanxi, Henan, Liaoning, and Beijing.

When the Guizhou Provincial Hygiene and Quarantine Prevention Station conducted a survey of endemic fluorosis caused by burning of coal in Guaier village of Guiyang City in 1989, 98.47% of children with 8-15 years old of age were found to have dental fluorosis and 72.79% of those over 16 exhibited functional impairment of joint movement, with a confirmed prevalence of skeletal fluorosis of 71.34%. From 1987 to 1989, the Chinese Ministry of Health launched similar surveys in Wushan, Qianjiang and Wulong counties in Sichuan Province, and Badong and Zigui counties in Hubei Province on the epidemic situation of coal burning type of endemic fluorosis. The results showed that the prevalence of skeletal fluorosis diagnosed by X-ray was as high as 57.2%, with 13.2% of these patients suffering from the disease more severe than degree II and 1-2% who had completely lost the ability to take care of themselves.

Currently, 13 provinces or regions in China are known to be affected by coal-burning type of endemic fluorosis, where mainly distributes in the mountainous areas in Southwestern of China and the regions of Yangtze River and Three Gorges. Severe endemic areas have been found in Guizhou, Yunnan, Sichuan, Chongqing, Hubei and Hunan provinces. Altogether, 173 counties (cities or districts) are affected by this type of endemic fluorosis, with 32.65 million people at risk, 14.537 million patients suffering from dental fluorosis, and 1.882 million from skeletal fluorosis.

3.2.1.3 Brick-tea Type of Endemic Fluorosis

Endemic fluorosis can also be caused by long-term excessive intake of fluoride present in brick tea, milk tea or oil tea, which contains high level of fluoride. This brick tea type of fluorosis, found only in China, was first identified in Tibetan regions of Sichuan Province in 1989. Although knowledge about this type of fluorosis is quite recent, epidemiological surveys have already made great progress.

Since the early 1980s, it has been confirmed that brick-tea type of endemic fluorosis prevails primarily in Sichuan, Xinjiang, Inner Mongolia, Gansu, Qinghai, and Tibet. Furthermore, the epidemic survey of 2006-2007 revealed that this disease did exist in Tibet, Sichuan, Inner Mongolia, Qinghai, Xinjiang, Gansu, and Ningxia, involving 316 counties and 3246 townships with a total population of 31 million. Most of these endemic areas are inhabited by Tibetans and the next largest number by Mongolians. In addition, the endemic areas severely affected by the disease are mainly distributed in the ethnic regions in Tibet, Sichuan and Gansu. In these areas, the average prevalence of dental fluorosis in children aged 8-12 years old was 20.5% and in adults 24.6%; the average prevalence of clinically diagnosed skeletal fluorosis of at least degree II in adults 12.6%; the average prevalence skeletal fluorosis diagnosed by X-ray in adults 32.1%. The findings indicated that dental fluorosis in children was relatively mild and skeletal fluorosis in adults relatively serious.

3.2.2　The Natural Causes of Endemic Fluorosis

3.2.2.1　Causes of Drinking Water Type of Endemic Fluorosis

Geology, geography, climate and water conservation are among the major factors that influence endemic fluorosis due to drinking water, which in China comes primarily from surface and ground water. The content of fluoride in this water is influenced by the geological formation; degree of leaching by weather; chemical composition of surface soil and runoff water; and precipitation and evaporation of water. The concentrations of fluoride in natural surface water vary greatly related with the fluoride content in rocks and soil in river beds and the solubility of this ion.

In arid or semi-arid areas, fluoride in water comes mainly from fluoride-rich waste or surface water in the low flat regions. During droughts, this water evaporates rapidly, causing massive accumulation of fluoride. This is how the regions affected by fluorosis come into being. The fluoride in underground water is derived primarily from volcanic activity, as well as weathering, erosion and/or dissolution of fluoride-rich rocks. The fluoride produced by volcanic activities accumulates in nearby areas and contaminates runoff water. Following weathering and migration, fluorine-rich rocks end up on low land, where they are dissolved and eroded by surface and/or underground water. Moreover, the high temperature deep in the earth, causes underground water to rise through fractures in the crust, dissolving and carrying the fluoride in granite, sedimentary strata, etc., to water in shallow sand zone and, ultimately, to the surface to form fluoride-rich springs. In addition, intake of fluoride is affected by weather, climate and the presence of other chemicals in water. During droughts and hot weather people drink more water consumption, which means that individuals increase fluoride intake. The chemical composition of water, especially its hardness and alkalinity, exerts certain impact on both the concentration of fluoride in water and its biological effects. In China, the fluoride level in drinking water in areas affected by this type of endemic fluorosis is usually higher than 2 mg/L and can even be as high as 20 mg/L (Fig. 3. 2).

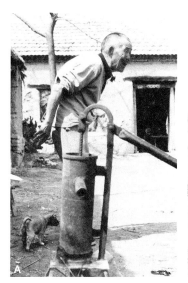
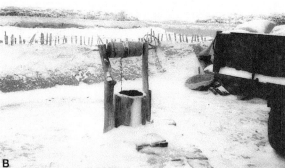

Fig. 3. 2   The source of high fluoride in water from areas of drinking water type of endemic fluorosis in China. A. A well with hand-pump; B. A windlass well.

3. 2. 2. 2   *Causes of Coal-burning Type of Endemic Fluorosis*

Natural environment, social economy and living habits are the three interwoven factors that influence the epidemic of endemic fluorosis caused by coal, which prevails mainly in the remote and cold highland areas of Southern China, where the high fluoride content of coal and soil is the major cause. In these areas, there is insufficient sunshine during the corn harvesting season to dry the corn, so the inhabitants have to do this drying by open burning of coal indoors. For the same reason in highland areas, the inhabitants usually dry chili and fresh vegetables for storage in the same manner. This procedure results in severe fluoride contamination of these major local foods since the mixture of coal and accompanying soil can contain as much as 1130 mg fluoride/kg. In addition, in winter the inhabitants use to keep warm by burning coal in open stove indoors because of the cold and wet weather (Fig. 3. 3), which also causes the fluoride contamination of the air. Thus, in such areas with severe coal-burning type of endemic fluorosis, the fluorine content on corn is 13. 5-130 mg/kg, on chili 82-940 mg/kg and in the air 0.1 mg/m^3. The long-

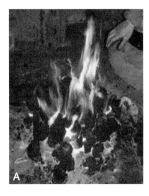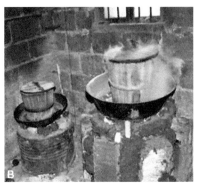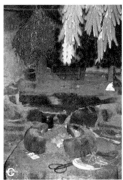

Fig. 3. 3   The source of high fluoride in endemic fluorosis area of coal-burning type.
A. Burning coal for warmth in winter; B. Cooking with open stove; C. Drying corn and chili
after harvest in autumn.

term consumption of fluorine-contaminated food and inhaling air with excessive fluoride leads to chronic fluorosis in humans.

3. 2. 2. 3   Causes of Brick-tea Type of Endemic Fluorosis

The ethnic inhabitants of western regions of China characterized by this type of endemic fluorosis are in the habit of drinking brick-tea, often made from fermented and pressed leafs and stems of coarse tea with a fluoride content usually greater than 300 mg/kg and as high as 1000 mg/kg. These groups consume large amounts of beef and lamb, and drink brick-tea to aid digestion, as well as to supplement vitamins, which are normally obtained from vegetables and fruits, but difficult to grow in these areas. Gradually, drinking brick-tea has become a part of everyday life, just as green tea has in other parts of China (Fig. 3. 4).

3. 2. 3   Do Social Factors Influence Endemic Fluorosis?

The development and occurrence of endemic fluorosis is influenced strongly by social factors such as local economy, culture, level of education, health, personal hygiene and diet, and is prevalent in areas with an underdeveloped economy, low living standard and malnutrition. For geographic, climatic and historical reasons, transportation and communication with the outside world is difficult in many such areas. Moreover, relatively scattered residences, poor health awareness and inadequate local health services further promote this endemic disease. Inhabitants

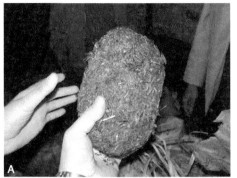
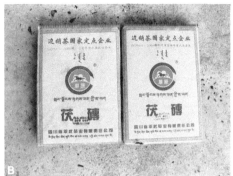
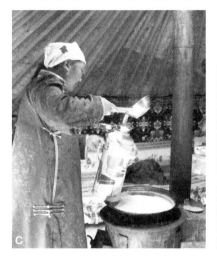
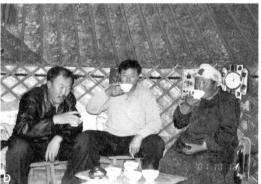

Fig. 3. 4　The source of high fluoride in tea in the brick-tea type of endemic fluorosis.
A and B. Brick-tea; C and D. Residents in the areas boiling and drinking brick-tea.

in these areas consume too few calories and too little protein, calcium and vitamins, which weakens their resistance against chronic fluorosis. Pregnant women and children, who need more nutrients are especially easy to suffer from malnutrition and chronic fluorosis.

With little knowledge on the risks of fluorosis, inhabitants in the areas with coal-burning type of fluorosis cook and dry food with open stoves indoor, and see no need for a chimney, resulting in severe fluorine pollution. In other regions, the ethnic population has quite a simple diet and drink large amounts of brick-tea every day, which is the main reason why they develop chronic fluorosis.

3.3 What Is Metabolic Pathway and Physiological Role of Fluoride in Our Body?

3.3.1 Metabolism

Following absorption via our digestive and respiratory tracts and skin, fluoride quickly enters in our circulation, with blood fluoride level rising significantly in only a few minutes, reaching the semi-absorbing phase after 30 minutes and peaking within 30-60 minutes. The soluble of fluoride, such as NaF tablets or in solution, may be absorbed completely, whereas fluoride with low solubility, such as CaF_2, MgF_2 and AlF_3 is difficult to be absorbed quickly or completely.

Uptake of fluoride, which is carried out by passive diffusion, occurs primarily in the stomach, where the high pH in gastric juice may result in the formation of uncharged hydrogen fluoride, which passes through the cell wall more rapidly than fluoride itself. Fluoride that is not absorbed in the stomach may be later absorbed in the small intestine in a pH-independent manner. In addition, the respiratory tract, skin and oral mucosa absorb small amounts of fluoride. On the other hand, the amounts of fluoride intaken from food depend on the solubility of inorganic fluoride, as well as the content of calcium in diet. Normally, 80% of the fluoride in food is taken up, but this value may go down to 50% if calcium or aluminum compound is present in the diet to form insoluble salts with the fluoride.

Human blood contains both free inorganic fluoride and bound organic fluoride, appoximately 75% of which exists in the plasma and the remainder in erythrocytes. Almost all serum fluoride is present as the anion, which does not bind to blood protein or other circulating components and has a half-life of 4-10 hours. The stability of serum fluoride depends on the dosage and frequency of intake. The fluoride content of breast milk is only half that of the serum, while the fluoride concentration in saliva is approximately 2/3 of the serum level, which may partially reflected the fluoride level of serum.

Due to its affinity for calcified tissues, 99% of the fluoride in the human body is present in the skeleton and teeth, where it binds with cryolite in the form of hydroxylapatite or fluorapatite. Fluoride that accumulates in the substantial spongiosa may later be released into the blood, and thereby represents a depot of fluoride. Fluoride can also cross the placenta and blood brain barriers. In addition, fluoride enters in the teeth during their formation, mineralization and post-mineralization, accumulating mainly on the enamel surface. During dental development, the average concentration of fluorine is 150 mg/kg in permanent enamel, but can as high as 2000 mg/kg in surface enamel of individuals who drink water with a desirable content of fluoride.

The kidney is the key organ that excretes fluoride, with 75% of fluoride excretes in the urine. The excreted content of fluoride in urine (usually < 1 mg/L) depends on the rate of glomerular filtration and 10-90% of the fluoride filtered may be reabsorbed by the nephric tubules. Chronic intake of fluoride may be in balance with the amount excreted in urine and deposited in bones, in which case the fluoride content of urine may reflect nearly the total intake. Therefore, the fluoride content in urine may be considered as an important indicator of excessive intake surveillance. Fluoride excreted through bowel movement accounts for 12.6-19.5% of the total; through sweat glands 7-10%; and through tear, hair, and fingernails much less.

3.3.2 Physiology

At appropriate levels, fluoride, a trace element in the human body, exerts certain biochemical metabolisms and physiological actions at suitable dosage. As mentioned above, fluoride accumulates in the skeleton and teeth, both rich in calcium and phosphorus, where it replaces the hydroxy in hydroxylapatite to form fluorapatite. In addition to improving the mechanical strength and acid resistance of these hard tissues, this stabilizes the calcium and phosphorus there. Suitable amount of fluoride may help maintain dental health and lack of the ion increase human susceptibility to dental caries. Thus, too much or too little fluoride may lead to a certain imbalance in calcium and phosphorus levels. However, due to the accessibility of fluoride in our environment, fluoride deficiency is uncommon.

3.4 Which Organs or Systems Are Impaired by Endemic Fluorosis?

Endemic fluorosis is a chronic disease that affects every part of the human body. In addition to the typical dental and skeletal fluorosis, excessive intake of fluoride may exert an impact on neurological, digestive, urinary, cardiovascular, and endocrinological systems, among others.

3. 4. 1　Dental Fluorosis

During dental development, excessive intake of fluoride leads to incomplete mineralization of enamel in association with decoloration of its surface in form of white flecks, brown staining and pitting, which is called dental fluorosis (Fig. 3. 5). Pathological alterations are usually observed in permanent teeth on both sides of the mouth, particularly the incisors followed by the molars, and upper teeth.

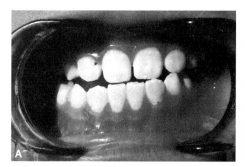
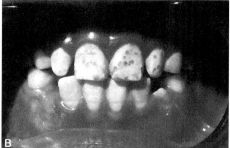
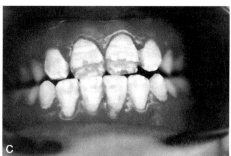

Fig. 3. 5　Dental fluorosis. A. Mild dental flourosis; B. Moderate dental fluorosis with small round pits in the opaque enamel; and C. Severe dental fluorosis where the enamel has been destroyed and there are large defective areas on several teeth.

3. 4. 1. 1　Clinical Manifestations

(1) Chalk-like alteration. The surface of the tooth enamel partially or completely loses its gloss, and epaque spots, stripes, or even the entire surface looks like chalk.

(2) Brown staining of the enamel. This change includes spots, stripes, or even

massive light browning, browning, dark browning, even black browning that cannot be removed.

(3) Enamel impairment. The enamel is destroyed, comes off or becomes spots, or covered with map-like pitting on the surface of teeth. This impairment is limited to enamel, not descending below the alveolar boundary. Large areas of impairment may be observed in severe cases.

3.4.1.2 The Major Underlying Mechanisms

(1) Fluoride affects the proliferation and differentiation of the cells that produce enamel, and thereby the synthesis and secretion of enamel matrix, resulting in morphological alteration of these cells.

(2) Fluoride easily replaces the hydroxy group in the hydroxylapatite in tooth enamel, transforming it into fluorapatite, as well as replacing the phosphate group. Ultimately, this forms insoluble calcium fluoride, which accumulates in growing teeth, prevents formation of the normal crystal structure of enamel, and produces an irregular structure, with local rough, staining, and other forms of impairment.

3.4.2 Skeletal Fluorosis

Another typical feature of endemic fluorosis is skeletal fluorosis (Fig.3.6), which usually appears after dental fluorosis as a manifestation of severe chronic fluorosis.

3.4.2.1 Clinical Manifestations

Skeletal fluorosis is usually observed in young adults and more cases have been reported in women. The primary clinical symptoms are pain in joints at waist and in the legs, rigid joints, bone malformation, and expression of nervous roots and of the spine. Patients often complain about constant pains in the spine and limb joints, which can be aggravated by remaining still and mitigated by exercise. No inflammatory manifestations such as congestion of blood vessels or swelling of joints have been observed. The pain is severe in patients with a pinched nerve root who usually refuse to be touched or help.

In severe cases joints or the spine may be immobilized. The spine bends laterally and humpback and rigid limbs are usually present, which may make life very

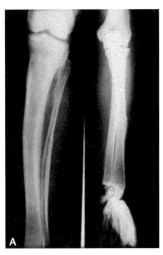
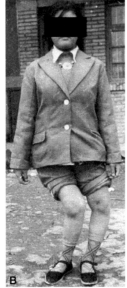
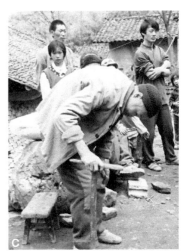

Fig. 3.6　Skeletal fluorosis. A. Alteration of the tibia observed by X-ray; B. Deformation of the legs; C. Deformation of the spinal column.

difficult. A compressed spine or nerve roots may lead to numbness and pain in the arms or legs; the whole body feels tied up and there may be limb paralysis, forcing the patient to stay bent over in bed, where coughing or turning may cause severe pain. These patients often demonstrate general muscular pain and atrophy, as well as alteration in their electrocardiograms (ECG).

3.4.2.2　Major Underlying Mechanisms

(1) Fluoride replaces the hydroxy group in the hydroxylapatite in bones and forms insoluble calcium fluoride that accumulates and affects the metabolism and structure of the bones. Bone malfunction is often observed by x-ray.

(2) Sclerosed, proliferated and deformed bone presses on the spine and nerve roots, resulting in numbness and pain in the limbs.

(3) The formation of insoluble calcium fluoride may decrease the level of calcium in the blood and stimulate the secretion of parathyrine, thereby causing resulting in abnormal metabolism of calcium and phosphorus.

(4) The impact of excessive fluoride on collagen metabolism in bone tissues may alter the quality of bone matrix. Disturbance of the regulation of bone

metabolism may cause proliferation and/or activation of osteoblasts, and accelerate bone transformation.

(5) Excessive fluoride impairs the functions of cartilage cells and stimulates proliferation of the periosteum and endosteum, resulting in the formation of new bone, as well as causing other morphological and functional alterations.

(6) Fluoride can bind to calcium and magnesium in the blood after being ingested, causing muscular spasm and pain. This can have bidirectional effects on bone metabolism, resulting in osteosclerosis, osteoporosis or osteomalacia alone, or a mixture of these types as a consequence of abnormal bone turnover.

3.4.3 Non-skeletal Impairment of Multiple Other Organs

Non-skeletal impairment due to endemic fluorosis is attracting more and more attention. Research in recent years indicates that the impairments of chronic fluorosis almost concern every systems or organs. Extensive research achievement has identified the nervous, urinary, digestive, cardiovascular and endocrine systems as the other major targets affected by chronic fluorosis.

Pathological alterations and metabolic disorders of the central nervous system caused by chronic fluorosis have attracted particularly much attention since fluoride can across the brain-blood barrier. Fluoride content in the brain tissues increases with more intake and high level of fluoride can produce histo-pathological changes, abnormalities in the cholinergic nervous system, structural alteration of the plasma-or bio-membrane of neurons, changes in receptors for neurotransmitters and alteration of signal transduction, among other effect. Interestingly, numerous epidemiological surveys indicate that the average intelligence quotient of children living in the areas with endemic fluorosis is significantly lower than normal.

Chronic fluorosis can also lead to morphological and functional abnormalities in the kidney, as seen in the altered ultrastructure of nephric tubule epithelial cells and an apparent impairment of renal functions.

The liver plays important role in detoxification and energy metabolism. Chronic fluorosis can cause morphological alterations, including degeneration of hepatocytes, appearance of a blurry border between liver cells, collapse of cellular organelles and swelling of mitochondria, among other things. Changes in liver function, including a reduced detoxifying capability have also been detected.

Moreover, apparent alterations in the ECG, conductibility and automaticity of myocardium, and lipid metabolism have also been observed in patients living in areas of endemic fluorosis. Investigations on animal models have revealed that the atherosclerosis associated with chronic fluorosis is related to disturbance of lipid metabolism.

Finally, the alterations in thyroid functional observed both in patients and experimental animals with endemic fluorosis include lower level of thyroxin and higher thyrotropin in the blood, and abnormal morphology of this organ such as significantly enlarged follicles.

3.4.4　Major Pathogenesis

The etiology and the cause of endemic fluorosis are clearly established. It is widely accepted both in China and international society of fluoride research, that long-term intake of excessive fluoride may induce deposition of this anion in the body and lead to extensive injury of multiple organs and systems. However, the pathogenesis of endemic fluorosis is extremely complicated and the mechanisms underlying whole-body toxicity remain elusive.

During the last century, many hypotheses concerning the mechanism underlying the general impairment caused by endemic or chronic fluorosis have been proposed, including alterations in protein, nucleic acids, enzyme activities, and abnormal collagen metabolism. However, since these alterations are observed only in certain organs or systems, none of these has gained widespread acceptance as an explanation for the systemic damage caused by the disease.

In the past 10 years, researchers have related the pathogenesis of endemic fluorosis primarily to an increased level of oxidative stress, alterations in signal transduction pathways, enhanced apoptosis, structural and functional modification of cell membrane, disturbance of calcium metabolism, mitochondrial changes, etc. Among these, oxidative stress has attracted the most attention.

Fluorine is a more active element which may cause cellular breathing breakout and the reactions involving free radicals. When excessive fluoride enters into the body, this anion can interfere with reactions involving oxygen and thereby elevate the level of oxygen free radicals, which react with a multitude compounds and destroy the normal structure and physiological function of tissues. The levels of reactive oxygen in many tissues of experimental animals with chronic fluorosis have been shown to be elevated by electron spin resonance. Moreover, chronic fluorosis affects trace elements which are involved in antioxidant activity, thereby reducing this activity and increasing the level of free radicals in this manner as well.

An elevated level of products of lipid peroxidation in the blood, the lower activity of antioxidant enzymes, such as superoxide dismutase (SOD), and elevated activities of peroxidase and catalase (which increase production of free radicals) are observed in patients living in areas with endemic fluorosis. In the tissues of experimental animals with chronic fluorosis and in cultured cells exposed to fluoride, the content of coenzyme Q, an endogenous antioxidant, was decreased. Interestingly, chronic fluorosis can decrease the expression of neuronal nicotinic acetylcholine receptors, which have been proved with anti oxidatant activity. The inhibited expression of the receptors may increase the level of oxidative stress, which in a way provides indirect evidence to prove the pathogenesis of chronic fluorosis induced by oxidative stress. Many reports have shown that chronic fluorosis alters the expression of mitochondrial fusion and fission proteins in many different organs, resulting in cellular injuries. The alterations indicated above emphasize that the increased level of oxidative stress could be one important mechanism in the pathogenesis of chronic fluorosis.

In recent years, most researchers in this area, both in China and internationally, have focused on treating endemic fluorosis with antioxidant(s). Vitamin E, vitamin C, selenium, catechuic nutgall acid, melatonine and others attenuate the elevated levels of lipid hyperoxides and organ injuries due to chronic fluorosis, providing a promising therapeutic approach in treating and preventing endemic fluorosis.

Apoptosis appears to play a central role in damages induced by endemic fluorosis. Recently, the abnormal expressions of many genes concerning apoptosis have been found to be related with the reduced activity of antioxidant enzymes or substances by chronic fluorosis. Apoptosis is considered to be the cause of extensive cell injury due to endemic fluorosis and increase level of oxidative stress may be the main inducer of apoptosis in the disease.

The many signal transduction pathways shown to be altered by chronic fluorosis include those involving mitogen-activated protein kinase (MAPK), phosphatidylinosital 3-kinase/protein kinase B (PI3-K/AKT) and advanced glycation end products and their receptor (AGEs/RAGE) pathways.

The major changes in abnormal lipid structures of bio-membranes have been found in the brain, liver and kidney of experiment animals with chronic fluorosis involve phospholipids, neutral lipids and polyunsaturated fatty acids. Since the normal structure of cellular bio-membranes is the foundation for maintaining the permeability, mobility, ion transport, receptor binding, and the activities of membrane enzymes, such structural abnormalities may be one cause of cellular injuries induced by chronic fluorosis. In addition, alterations in calcium homeostasis, energy metabolism, gene polymorphism, etc. also demonstrate apparent correlations with the development of endemic fluorosis, which may be an important part in the pathogenesis of systemic impairments caused by the disease.

3.5 Can Endemic Fluorosis Be Diagnosed Clinically?

3.5.1 Clinical Diagnosis of Dental Fluorosis

The WHO has recommended that dental fluorosis be diagnosed employing the index devised by Dean in 1934, and revised in 1935, 1938 and 1942. Dean's index scores dental fluorosis as questionable, very mild, mild, moderate and severe fluorosis (total 5 degrees), which is simple, convenient, reproducible and suitable for large-scale epidemiological surveys.

Since the regions of endemic fluorosis in China are widely distributed and the situations are complicated, the diagnostic criteria utilized must be clear, simple and easily applied. Therefore, the Chinese diagnostic criteria for dental fluorosis (WT/T208-2011), a modification of the Dean's index, grades dental fluorosis as normal (i. e., none), questionable, very mild, mild, moderate, and severe; remove the confusing and inappropriate parts of the Dean's index; and clarify every level in detail. These criteria have proven to be quite valuable in China.

3.5.2　Clinical Diagnosis of Skeletal Fluorosis

The diagnosis of skeletal fluorosis in areas of endemic fluorosis must fulfill the following requirements: (1) the patients must have been living in region and have a history of excessive fluoride intake; (2) show signs of dental fluorosis (individuals migrating into the area after reaching adulthood may be exempted from this), accompanied with joint pain, limitation of movement, and even deformed limbs; (3) exhibit a fluoride level in the urine that is higher; (4) show symptoms upon a X-ray examination of osteosclerosis, osteoporosis and/or osteomalacia (bone transformation), periosteum and joint deformation.

　　Based on the pain in the body and joints, the degree of dyskinesia and the X-ray examinations, skeletal fluorosis can be categorized as mild, moderate or severe. The X-ray examination should be given priority as compared to manifestations when these two tests are controversy. This diagnosis should discriminate between skeletal fluorosis and bone arthritis, rheumatic arthritis, ankylosing spondylitis and rheumatoid arthritis.

3.5.3　Related Diagnostic Indicators in the Laboratory

Laboratory indicators play an important complementary role, not only in early diagnosis before apparent skeletal fluorosis develops, but also in assessing the effectiveness of prevention and treatment of the disease. Although much research on laboratory indicators of early stages of fluorosis has been conducted both in China and internationally, and valuable results obtained, more works in this area are still required.

3.5.3.1　Fluoride Content

The fluoride content in tissues and organs is usually related closely to the extent of pathological impairment. With the availability of more assays and improvement of their sensitivity, fluoride content in various tissues and/or in the urine may aid early diagnosis of chronic fluorosis.

　　Blood The fluoride level in serum (or plasma) is correlated to intake and excretion of this anion. Prior to a meal, the blood level of fluoride parallels the urinary level and is somewhat affected by renal function, making this valuable indicator in early diagnosis of chronic fluorosis. The blood levels of inhabitants in areas of endemic fluorosis are generally higher than those in non-fluorosis areas, but this level in blood fluoride content in the patients with skeletal fluorosis may not be higher than in those patients without skeletal fluorosis. Therefore, the fluoride content in the blood can serve as an indicator for populations exposed to excessive fluoride, but only as a reference for individual values.

Urine In general, the urinary level of fluoride is lower than 1 mg/L in non-fluorosis areas, and higher than 2 mg/L and even as high as 10 mg/L in regions of endemic fluorosis. Elevated excretion of fluoride in the urine usually indicates excessive intake or the presence of accumulated fluoride. To some extent the blood and urinary level of fluoride are positively correlated, objectively reflecting the degree of fluorosis. The level of fluoride in the urine is a reliable indicator of the diagnosis for endemic fluorosis, a valuable tool for following progression of chronic fluorosis, and helpful to a certain extent in early diagnosis of individual chronic fluorosis.

Other possibility The fluoride contents of bone, fingernails and hair are all sometimes used as indicators of endemic fluorosis. Since most of ingested fluoride accumulates in bones, the level of the anion there may accurately reflect whole body accumulation. Clinically, however, bone samples are too difficult to be obtained as a regular indicator in this context. In addition, fingernails and hair are easy to be obtained as biological samples, but no significant differences between the fluoride content of the hair from the individuals living in regions of endemic fluorosis and other areas have been detected.

3. 5. 3. 2 Biomarkers

Biomarkers are biological indicators with the capability of recording the structural or functional alterations of the systems, organs, tissues, cells and subcellular structures, which subjects to wide applications.

Serum enzymology Routine biochemical assays of enzyme activities, the protein content, electrolyte concentrations, etc. in the blood are important biomarkers for endemic fluorosis. The levels of enzyme activities and other factors related to oxidative stress in a variety of tissues and organs, including the blood, of individuals with endemic fluorosis are abnormal, e.g., the clearly lowered activities of SOD and glutathione peroxidase (GSH-Px), the reduced total antioxidant capacity of blood, and the elevated circulating level of malondialdehyde (MDA). Recently, the activities of myeloperoxidase (MPO) and GSH-Px have been found to be significantly higher in people living in areas of coal-burning type of endemic fluorosis than those in non-fluorosis areas. Serum alkaline phosphatase is an important indicator for assessing bone formation and transformation during the progression of skeletal fluorosis, and can serve as a sensitive marker for early diagnosis of endemic fluorosis.

Hormones related to regulation of metabolism Endemic fluorosis has a significant impact on the functions of thyroid gland, manifested by the antagonism between fluorine and iodine. Fluoride can influence the uptake and utilization of iodine by the thyroid gland and thereby decrease the synthesis of thyroxine. The lowered thyroxine level in the blood of patients living in regions with endemic fluorosis is accompanied by mild thyroid hypofunction and enhanced secretion of parathyrine.

Alterations in blood-fat The total cholesterol and triglyceride levels in blood are clearly elevated in patients with skeletal fluorosis in regions of endemic fluorosis, while the level of high-density lipoprotein is significantly reduced. These three levels can be used in early diagnosis.

Relevant indicators in the urine Elevated level of creatinine and total urea nitorgen in urine can serve as an early indicator of renal impairment caused by endemic fluorosis. In addition, alteration of the calcium and phosphate levels in urine may indirectly reflect a change in the homeostasis of these ions.

3.6 Characterization of the Different Regions of Endemic Fluorosis

3.6.1 Endemic Fluorosis Area of Drinking Water Type

The fluoride content in the drinking water of the village is more than 1.2 mg/L and the prevalence of dental fluorosis among children aged 8-12 and who were born and live in the area is greater than 30%.

3.6.2 Endemic Fluorosis Area of Coal-burning Type

The prevalence of dental fluorosis among children aged 8-12 and who were born and live in the area is greater than 30%.

3.6.3 Endemic Fluorosis Area of Brick-tea Type

In the population older than 16 years old, the average amount of fluoride taken in daily by drinking brick tea is more than 3.5 mg and there are patients with skeletal fluorosis as confirmed by X-ray examination.

3.7 Definition of Regions with Endemic Fluorosis and Different Degrees of Severity

3.7.1 Endemic Fluorosis Area of Drinking Water or Coal-Burning Type

3.7.1.1 Regions of Mild Endemic Fluorosis

The prevalence of moderate and severe dental fluorosis among children aged 8-12 and born and living in the area is ≤20%, or the patients with skeletal fluorosis confirmed by X-ray examination have only mild, no moderate or serious disease.

3.7.1.2 Regions of Moderate Endemic Fluorosis

The prevalence of moderate and severe dental fluorosis among children aged 8-12 and born and living in the area is 20-40% or ≤2% of the patients with skeletal fluorosis confirmed by X-ray examination, are afflicted by the severe form of the disease.

3.7.1.3 Regions of Severe Endemic Fluorosis

The prevalence of moderate and severe dental fluorosis among children aged 8-12 and born and living in the area is more than 40%, or >2% of the patients with skeletal fluorosis confirmed by X-ray examination suffer from the severe form of this disease.

3.7.2 Endemic Fluorosis Area of Brick-tea Type

3.7.2.1 Regions of Mild Endemic Fluorosis

There are no patients aged 36-45 with moderate or severe skeletal fluorosis, as determined by X-ray.

3. 7. 2. 2   Regions of Moderate Endemic Fluorosis

The prevalence of moderate or severe skeletal fluorosis among patients aged 36-45, as determined by X-ray, is no more than 10%.

3. 7. 2. 3   Regions of Severe Endemic Fluorosis

The prevalence of moderate or severe skeletal fluorosis among patients aged 36-45 is greater than 10%, as determined by X-ray.

3. 8   Prevention and Control of Endemic Fluorosis

For an endemic disease like fluorosis, prevention and control are more important than treatment. In addition to reducing the amount of fluoride ingested, reducing the absorption of ingested fluoride, stimulating fluoride excretion and balanced nutrition should be encouraged.

3. 8. 1   What Measures for the Control and Prevention of Endemic Fluorosis Caused by Drinking Water Are Available?

The basic effective measure for controlling endemic fluorosis associated with drinking water is to reduce the fluoride content of the water in accordance with established hygienic criteria—either monitoring the fluoride content by changing water source and/or defluoridation of drinking water.

3. 8. 1. 1   Changing to Low-fluoride Water

The first choice is to look for a source of water with a low fluoride content, commonly used deep groundwater, surface water uncontaminated by natural sources of fluoride, and/or rainfall. Thus, obtaining supplies of low-fluoride water usually involves installation of deep water wells at appropriate locations, extraction of low-fluoride surface water (e.g. from rivers, lakes and springs), harvesting and storing rain water, and, if necessary, mixing high-and low-fluoride water to achieve an acceptable level. In China, the construction of deep water wells into low-fluoride aquifers is the main preventive measure initiated by the government(Fig. 3. 7).

The fluoride content of deep groundwater in areas with high-fluoride shallow groundwater is generally low and suitable for drinking. However, the following should be taken into consideration when exploiting deep groundwater: (1) Prior to

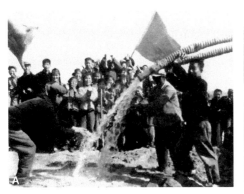
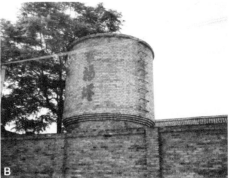

Fig. 3. 7 Projects designed to improve the quality of drinking water. A. The first low-fluoride water well in China designed to prevent fluorosis caused by drinking water in Qian' an County, Jilin Province; B. Improved water supply apparatus in Shandong province.

drilling, an appropriate geological agency must be consulted to confirm the results of groundwater quality analyses and the proposed drilling depth. (2) During and after construction, the water wells must be sealed completely to avoid surface contamination and interaction with shallow groundwater. (3) Once the well is established at the intended depth, checking and acceptance criteria must be strictly observed to ensure that the fluoride content in the water fulfills quality criteria. (4) The water quality must be monitored continuously and long-term.

If there is a naturally occurring source of low-fluoride surface water near an area affected by fluorosis, a channel or pipeline can deliver the water where it is needed. If the supply of low-fluoride water is inadequate to meet the demand, then this water can be combined with high-fluoride water to obtain a mixture that still complies with hygienic criteria. If there is no source of low-fluoride water, small reservoirs or cisterns can be utilized to collect rainfall and snow (Fig. 3. 8). No matter what the source of the water, the basic requirement is to provide a reliable and sufficient quantity of water that conforms with recognized hygienic standards.

3. 8. 1. 2   Defluoridation of Drinking Water

Prevention and control of fluorosis through improvement of the water supply is difficult, requiring appropriate knowledge, technology, organization, engineering, and funding. Where conversion to a source of low-fluoride water is not possible, defluoridation of high-fluoride drinking water by physical and/or chemical methods is

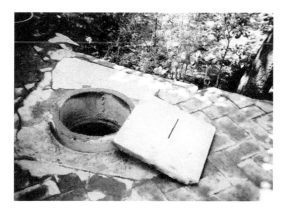

Fig. 3. 8　Cistern used to collect rainfall and snow in the Gansu Province.

the only measure for preventing fluorosis. However, many different procedures for defluoridation have been developed and choosing one that is appropriate for each particular situation is extremely important for satisfactory performance.

In developing countries, common defluoridation methods include coagulation and precipitation with aluminum salt, adsorption by activated alumina, and filtration through hydroxyapatite, bone charcoal or clay. A flow chart for simple adsorption of fluoride is depicted in Fig. 3. 9. Coagulants commonly used in connection with the coagulant-sedimentation procedure are aluminum sulfate, aluminum chloride, and alkaline aluminum chloride; while with adsorption method include activated aluminum oxide and bone charcoal are commonly used. All of these substances have a hydroxyl metal network that facilitates exchanges other ions for fluoride.

Particle of activated aluminum (Al_2O_3) has adsorptive surface where pollutants and other substances in water flowing over it are retained. When exposed to water, bone charcoal, a black, porous granular material consisting of 57-80% calcium phosphate, 6-10% calcium carbonate and 7-10% active carbon, can absorb a large variety of pollutants including pigments as well as compounds responsible for taste and odor. In addition, because it is composed predominately of hydroxyl apatite ($Ca_{10}(PO_4)_6(OH)_2$), in which one or both OH^- ions can be replaced by F^-, bone charcoal possess a special capacity to absorb fluoride from water, allowing contact defluoridation.

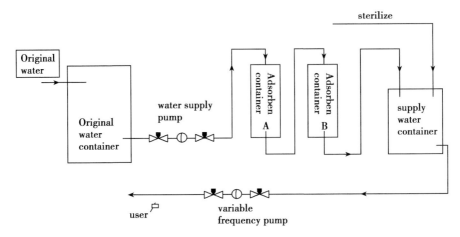

Fig. 3. 9   A flow chart for simple adsorption of fluoride.

Clay is a composed predominantly of particles of hydrous aluminum silicate and other minerals and impurities. When damp, clay has good texture and plasticity and it keeps its shape upon drying and forms a very hard sinter after being burned. Burnt clay and clay powder can adsorb fluoride and other pollutants from water. Clay powder can also clarify turbid water, a characteristic that the ancient Egyptians applied in their homes.

To date, several large-scale projects for defluoridation of drinking water have been put into operation (Fig. 3. 10).

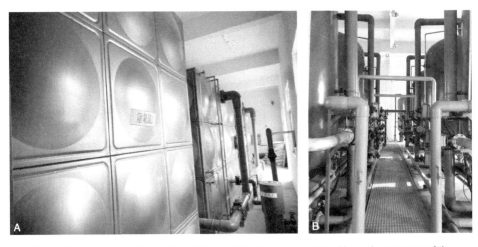

Fig. 3. 10   Apparatus for defluoridation of drinking water.A. In Mengcheng town of the Anhui Province; B. In Sanyi county of the Anhui Province.

More advanced technologies for defluoridation include electrodialysis, agglutination, reverse osmosis, ionization and distillation (Fig. 3. 11). The method of defluoridation should be appropriate for local conditions and water quality. For example, in areas where the water supply is scattered, units for physical and/or chemical defluoridation of drinking water can be set up in a village or even in an individual household.

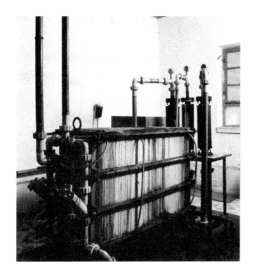

Fig. 3. 11 An electrodialyzer used for defluoridation of drinking water.

3. 8. 2 Measures for Control and Prevention of Endemic Fluorosis Caused by Burning Coal

Endemic fluorosis caused by pollution from burning coal is managed by comprehensive prevention based both on health education and the use of more efficient stoves.

3. 8. 2. 1 More efficient Stoves

To reduce the amount of smoke containing fluoride that arises from the burning of coal in households, which is inhaled and contaminates foods, better stoves that effectively release smoke outdoor are required. Furthermore, through scientific design, such stoves can combust coal more efficiently, thereby reducing both coal consumption and the total emission of fluoride. In addition, other measures such as purification and fixation of fluoride and sulfur can be implemented. The basic requirements of a stove designed to reduce fluoride emissions are reliability, safety and sanitation, efficiency, economy and practicality, sturdiness and durability. Fig. 3. 12 illustrates the design of such an improved coal-burning stove.

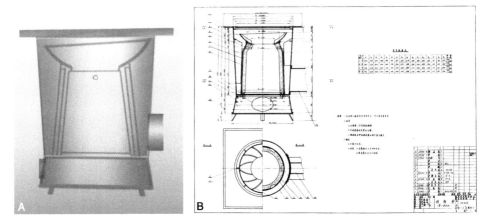

Fig. 3. 12　The design of an improved coal-burning stove. A. Overall appearance; B. Internal lay-out.

3. 8. 2. 2　Reducing or Eliminating Pollution of Food by Fluoride

In regions with endemic fluorosis due to coal burning, most intake of fluoride by the residents is in the form of contaminated food, especially pepper, which together with corn, they hang directly above the stove to dry. Furthermore, food sanitation in these areas is very poor, typically, peppers are eaten unwashed, resulting in a fluoride intake that greatly exceeds the recommended.

Therefore, reducing fluoride pollution through food requires more than simply use of improved stoves. Implementation of such technology must be supplemented with health education, raising awareness, guidance and encouragement of local residents to cultivate, harvest, dry and store crops in an appropriate manner. These efforts should be incorporated into coordinated campaigns designed to improve food hygiene, raise consciousness about prevention of disease and cultivate good living habits that promote health.

Appropriate actions of this sort include the followings: (1) Advocate the use of mulch in cultivating crops and/or changing the manner of planting so that crops mature more rapidly and utilize available sunlight more effectively, thereby improving harvests. (2) Prevent foods from coming into direct contact with smoke during drying by flue-curing in a tobacco chamber instead, and avoid hanging food for long periods over the kitchen stove. (3) Hang preserved meat, after it has been pickled and smoked with firewood, somewhere in the house where it will not be exposed to smoke from burning coal. (4) After being dried, foodstuffs such as peppers and corn should be kept in sealed containers to reduce the chance of fluoride pollution. Dry lime can be added to these containers as a desiccant to prevent mildew and infestation by pests (e.g., moths and other insects).

3.8.2.3 Improving the Conditions and Layout of Housing

As part of health education, residents should be encouraged to take measures that preserve heat, such as tightening walls, doors and windows, thereby reducing coal consumption and the total output of pollutants. Furthermore, the bedroom should be some distance from the kitchen and ventilation should be adequate.

3.8.2.4 Additional Measures

Other measures designed to alleviate endemic fluorosis caused by burning coal include adopting more healthy living habits, such as washing grains prior to cooking, avoiding consumption of dust chili and over toasted chili, and using cleaner fuels (e. g., marsh gas, straw gas, etc.). If possible, a rice cooker, induction cooker, and electric heater should be used. In summary, the basic measures for alleviating endemic fluorosis caused by burning coal involve promoting economic development, improving the standard of living, and increasing the consciousness of disease prevention, to encourage local residents to abandon their old habit of burning coal in open stoves (Fig. 3.13).

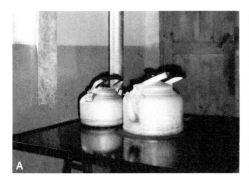
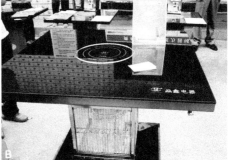

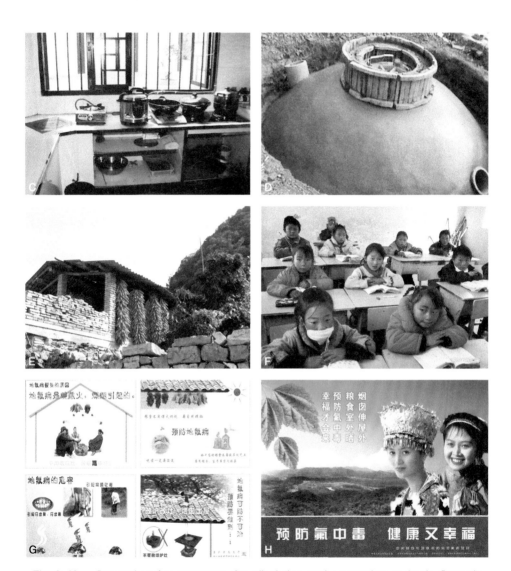

Fig. 3. 13 Comprehensive measures for alleviating and preventing endemic fluorosis caused by burning coal. A. An improved stove, with lid and chimney leading out of the house. B and C. A cookers and electromagnetic oven that use clean energy. D. A biogas digester for life fuel. E. Drying corns outside in the sunshine. F. Health education about endemic fluorosis in primary school. G to H. Wall posters promoting health education.

3. 8. 3 Alleviating and Preventing Brick-tea Type of Endemic Fluorosis

Since brick tea is an essential component of the diet of minority residents in the western regions of China, reduction of fluoride content in brick tea is of fundamental importance in this context. China's Fluoride Content of Brick Tea (GB19965-2005), the first national health standard of its kind in the world, requires that this content be no more than 300 mg/kg (300 ppm). At present, the Chinese government is actively encouraging tea manufacturers to change their production of brick tea to lower the fluoride content. However, most brick tea cannot currently meet the hygienic standard set for fluoride, so other comprehensive measures designed to reduce the intake of fluoride are also necessary.

3. 8. 3. 1 Defluoridation of Tea

Tea can be effectively defluoridated by washing it briefly in boiling water and then discarding this water prior to brewing. Since smaller particles have a greater surface area per mass than larger particles, more fluoride can be removed from small particles of tea in this manner, so the brick tea should be broken into smaller pieces prior to this washing. 65% or more of the fluoride in brick tea can be removed in this manner.

3. 8. 3. 2 Health Education Designed to Change the habit of Drinking Brick-tea

Health education should raise awareness and encourage residents to drink less high-fluoride brick tea. Instead, they should choose black tea, with a color, smell and taste similar to that of brick tea, but a lower content of fluoride. In addition, using milk tea instead or reducing the time for which brick tea is boiled can effectively decrease the amount of fluoride ingested.

3. 8. 3. 3 Improving Nutrition

Calcium, protein and vitamins can all counteract fluoride uptake by the body and promote fluoride excretion. Therefore, it is important to increase the intake of meat, dairy products, vegetables, and fruits by residents in regions of endemic fluorosis.

3. 8. 3. 4 Developing the Local Economy

To a certain extent, endemic disease is due to poverty, so that developing the local economy is an essential and important step. On the one hand, favorable economic conditions can alleviate exposure to causes of endemic disease. And on the other hand, better economic conditions can improve local lifestyle and living habits, raise the standard of living, improve nutrition, and enhance the ability to avoid disease. The role of economic development in disease prevention should not be underestimated.

3.9　Can Endemic Fluorosis Be Treated?

Although excess fluoride can accumulate in many different organs and lead to damage of different degrees, making treatment complex, the most common and serious damage caused by endemic fluorosis is to hard tissue, with the typical clinical manifestations being dental fluorosis and skeletal fluorosis.

3.9.1　Treatment of Dental Fluorosis

Once it has developed, dental fluorosis lasts a lifetime, so treatment is designed primarily to alleviate symptoms and improve appearance, as well as in the case of severe dental fluorosis, restore function. At present, clinical treatment involves bleaching and repair, individually or in combination. However, such treatment does not fundamentally solve the problem and the focus should be on prevention in the manner described above.

3.9.2　Treatment of Skeletal Fluorosis

There are no ideal procedures or medications for treatment of skeletal fluorosis. The medications employed include calcium, vitamin D, vitamin C, aluminum hydroxide, the Congrong Pill, the Gulingtongbi Pill, and hyperostosis pill, while clinical therapy is usually limited to symptomatic treatment designed to alleviate pain. Furthermore, improving nutrition can enhance fluoride excretion from the body.

In severe cases, skeletal fluorosis can cause serious joint deformity that limits a patient's ability to work or his/her quality of life due to symptoms caused by intervertebral foramen and canalis vertebralis stenosis (including paresthesia, intense pain, limited range of motion, and even incontinence and paralysis). In such cases, surgery should be considered, including joint orthotics, decompression of vertebral lamina and orthotics involving cutting of spinal bone.

3. 10　History of Control of Endemic Fluorosis in China

3. 10. 1　1960-1985: From Scattered Surveys That Identify the Nature and Distribution of the Disease to Implementation and Promotion of Pilot Programs for Changing to Low-fluoride Water Supplies

Prior to 1979, endemic fluorosis was not included in China's central program for the prevention and control of endemic disease, and no effective measures had been undertaken. Tentative efforts to change water supplies and decrease fluoride ingestion carried out only in parts of the provinces experiencing serious endemic fluorosis provided a certain amount of experience. After 1979, pilot programs to change supplies of water to other with lower fluoride content were carried out sequentially in various regions with fluorosis across the country, and achieving initial success.

In 1981, more than 1,000 electromechanical deep wells designed to provide low-fluoride groundwater were built in Baicheng City of Jilin Province, gradually replacing hand-pumped wells. In 1982, a working group in Shandong Province initiated a three-year pilot project designed to developing alternative low-fluoride water supplies in Gaomi County,and by the end of 1984, the progress made by this project was the fastest among such programs in China. From 1981 to 1984, projects designed to develop low-fluoride water supplies improved the situation for approximately 6,040,000 people throughout China.

3. 10. 2　1986-2006: Systematic and Standardized Prevention and Control of Endemic Fluorosis

3. 10. 2. 1　Widespread Recognition of the Importance of Reducing the Fluoride Content of Water Supplies

In September of 1989, the *Notification for Establishing Key National Surveillance Sites* for endemic fluorosis was issued by the Chinese Ministry of Health,and in 1991, surveillance began in certain key areas. The results showed that changing to low-fluoride water supplies significantly reduced the numbers of both areas of serious fluorosis and severely affected patients, confirming the effectiveness of this approach. To achieve long-term effects and consolidate them, the surveillance indicated that supplies of low-fluoride drinking water must become the standard for water engineering projects and their routine operation.

3. 10. 2. 2　Organization and Implementation of Pilot Projects to Control Endemic Fluorosis Resulting from Burning Coal: the Foundation for Full Implementation of These Measures

In 1987-1989, the Chinese Ministry of Health and the Ministry of Agriculture, Husbandry and Fisheries called upon the Chinese Center for Endemic Disease Control, the Chinese Academy of Preventive Medicine and Harbin Medical University to investigate the control of endemic fluorosis caused by pollution from burning coal. In a project lasting three years and involving 60 experts, professors and other researchers were dispatched to Wushan County, Qianjiang County and Wulong County of the Three Gorges area and to Badong County and Zigui County of Hubei Province to improve coal burning technology to reduce fluoride pollution. This study systematically revealed numerous scientific problems concerning with endemic fluorosis, including removing the source of fluoride pollution, characteristics of the disease and key measures for prevention and control.

This project led to the design, optimization and promotion of more than 10 types of coal-burning stoves (ovens), suitable for use in mountainous areas of different altitudes, as well as to identification of different types of coal and uses for the stoves (heating or cooking). The stoves of 150,000 families were improved in three years and, thereby, 630, 000 people protected from high fluoride intake. The pilot stove project in the Three Gorges area laid a solid technological foundation for controlling and further research on endemic fluorosis caused by burning coal in China (Fig. 3. 14).

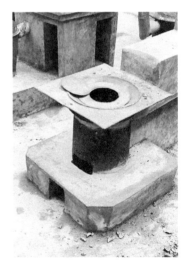

Fig. 3. 14　An improved stove, referred to as Wulong No. 1, being developed as a result of the pilot project.

3. 10. 2. 3   Assessing the Extent of Developing Low-fluoride Criteria, Providing
                Technical Support for Measures Designed to Combat Fluorosis Due to
                Drinking Brick-tea

From 1999 to 2006, China's leaders focused much attention on fluorosis caused by drinking brick tea. Many research institutions began to explore epidemiology, pathogenesis, contributing factors and measures to control this type of fluorosis. The main conclusions arrived at were as follows: (a) Fluorosis due to drinking brick tea was widely prevalent in the western areas of China populated by minority groups. (b) In areas affected by this type of fluorosis, adult intake of fluoride, more than 90% of which was in the form of brick tea, far exceeded the recommended standard. (c) Adult skeletal fluorosis, mostly in the form of osteoarthropathy was more severe in these areas than in those where fluorosis due to high-fluoride drinking water was prevalent. (d) Prevalence of the skeletal fluorosis elevated with age, with 40 years old representing an important turning point after which the prevalence increased significantly.

At the beginning of 2006, *the Fluoride Content of Brick Tea (GB19965-2005)* formulated official standard to be implemented by the Chinese government, designed to prevent and control fluorosis caused by drinking brick tea. At the end of this year, the central government allocated funds specifically for conducting a cross-sectional survey of the prevalence of this type of fluorosis in eight provinces, thereby clarifying for the first time the distribution and seriousness of the disease, as well as the dose-response relationship between fluorosis and intake of brick-tea, which is the basic detailed information required for targeting effective prevention and control measures at specific geographic regions.

To date, in the areas where fluorosis is attributed to the consumption of brick tea, targeted large-scale measures for prevention have not yet been implemented, but some institutions have conducted pilot projects designed to promote the use of low-fluoride brick tea. Such measures, along with economic progress are expected to effectively alleviate this type of fluorosis.

3. 10. 3 2007-2015: Control of Endemic Fluorosis Reaches a Crucial Stage

3. 10. 3. 1 Full Implementation of the Safe Drinking Water Project

The Chinese government attaches great importance to the problem of safe drinking water in rural areas. From 2002 to 2003, the National Development and Reform Commission included water improvement for the control of endemic disease in its list of projects to be funded by national bonds. The Ministry of Health called upon the Chinese Center for Endemic Disease Control and other departments involved develop a plan for water improvement for control of endemic disease in western regions and the Ministry of Water Resources carried out the work. Investment in this project totaled 850 million yuan and a significant portion of the population (56.18 million people) was benefited.

In January of 2007, the State Council approved and issued the *Eleventh National Five-year Plan for Engineering of safe Drinking Water in Rural Areas.* By the end of 2010, the problems with drinking water safety in the areas identified as moderately and severely affected by fluorosis were essentially solved. The subsequent Twelfth Five-year Plan of the government included engineering of safe drinking water in rural areas as one of the important elements of socialist development of new countryside and continued investment in relevant projects in all areas known to be affected by fluorosis. The implementation of this plan sped up water improvement in these areas considerably, and as a result, their drinking water is now essentially safe.

3. 10. 3. 2 Allocating Funds Specifically for the Prevention and Control of Endemic Disease; Full Implementation of Measures Designed to Improve Stoves in Areas Affected by Fluorosis Due to Burning Coal

Beginning in 2004, the Chinese government has provided central subsidies to control fluorosis caused by burning coal for local public health funds designed. In 10 provinces (Guizhou, Hubei, Hunan, Sichuan, Yunnan, Chongqing, Shaanxi, Jiangxi, Guangxi and Henan) comprehensive prevention and control was undertaken, including a baseline survey concerning the areas affected, improvement of stoves, and education about and promotion of health. In 2009, the Central Committee of the Communist Party of China issued *Opinions of the State Council on Deepening the Healthcare System*

Reform, including recommendations to reform major public health projects by including measures to control fluorosis caused by pollution from burning coal.

From 2004 to 2012, special funds amounting to 1.74 billion yuan (RMB) were invested in the improvement of stoves. In addition, all local levels of governments supplemented these funds significantly and national programs to improve stoves encompassed 5.17 million households, which combined with mass spontaneous adoption of improved stoves, resulted in 6.32 million families nationwide with new stoves. The proportion of households with improved stoves rose from 25.4% at the beginning of the project to 98.32% at present, i.e., this measure now has been implemented completely in all areas affected by fluorosis due to pollution from burning coal (Fig. 3. 15).

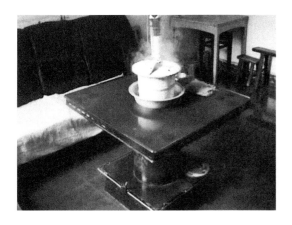

Fig. 3. 15 A new stove presently used in areas of endemic fluorosis of coal-burning type.

3. 11 The Achievements of China's Programs for Prevention and Control of Endemic Fluorosis

3. 11. 1 Disease Control Status

When national surveillance of endemic fluorosis began in 1991, the prevalence of dental fluorosis among children in areas where fluorosis was caused by high-fluoride drinking water was 60.08%. As a result of improvements in water supplies, this prevalence declined or tended to decline annually, falling to 20.61% by 2006. In 2007, surveillance at new locations resulted in an apparently higher rate of dental fluorosis in children than in 2006. After 2009, this prevalence has remained at approximately 25% or less. In comparison, in areas where fluorosis was caused by pollution from burning coal the locations of surveillance has changed more frequently and detection of dental fluorosis in children varied more widely.

A cohort study was designed to analyze skeletal fluorosis due to high-fluoride drinking water during four successive 5-year periods. As more time passed after making improvements in water supplies, the overall detection of skeletal fluorosis, either clinically or by X-ray, was higher exhibited a downward trend at all locations surveyed (Fig. 3. 16). In regions with fluorosis due to burning coal, the number of surveillance locations was lower and shifted more frequently, so that, the effect of stove improvements on the prevalence of skeletal fluorosis was not clear.

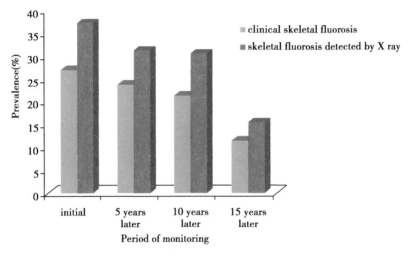

Fig. 3. 16   Detection of skeletal fluorosis during successive 5-year periods after making improvements in water supplies.

3. 11. 2   Research on and Control of Endemic Fluorosis Caused by Burning Coal or Drinking Brick-tea

Although efforts in China to control endemic fluorosis due to pollution from burning coal or drinking brick tea began later than those in areas affected by poor water quality, the results have been significant. In the 1980's, a pilot project implemented by the Chinese government in the Yangtze River Three Gorges region demonstrated that reducing fluoride emissions from stoves was an effective approach to alleviating endemic fluorosis due to pollution from burning coal. In addition, this project provided experience in the organization and management of project designed to change people's habits, as well as a scientific basis for future improvement of stoves, winning the second prize in the 1992 *National Award for Scientific and Technological Progress.*

In 1999, the Center for Endemic Disease Control of Chinese Center for Disease Control and Prevention promoted research on the prevalence of fluorosis caused by drinking brick tea and the relationship between intake of brick-tea and fluorosis in Sichuan and Inner Mongolia. A 10-year research project on the mechanisms underlying fluorosis and control measures was also launched. In 2006, utilizing central subsidies for support of local projects, each province concerned conducted an epidemiological survey of fluorosis arising from drinking brick tea. On the basis of the various efforts described above, the criteria for *Fluoride Content of Brick Tea* were developed, and the prevalence, severity, epidemiology, the mechanisms underlying this type of fluorosis characterized, and guidelines for prevention and control developed. In 2011, this project won second prize *in the Scientific and Technological Progress Award* from the Ministry of Education and second prize *in the Medical Scientific and Technological Award* from the Chinese Medical Association.

3. 11. 3 Standard System Development

From 1996 to 2001, a series of national health industrial criteria related to endemic fluorosis were issued and implemented. These included criteria for measurement of fluoride content and the normal range expected in various types of samples (such as urine, coal, and soil), as well as for medical decision, such as diagnosis of skeletal fluorosis and dental fluorosis. In addition, these criteria defined areas of endemic fluorosis and addressed control in these areas.

In 2006,standard of *Fluoride Content of Brick-Tea* was issued. Soon thereafter, the criteria for identification and categorization of areas of endemic fluorosis were revised to include fluorosis due to drinking brick tea. The diagnostic criteria for skeletal fluorosis and dental fluorosis were also revised in 2008 and 2011, respectively. In 2015, to adapt to the need of preventing and controlling fluorosis arising from burning coal, as well as to evaluate effects objectively and scientifically in a standardized manner, appropriate criteria were formulated. As indicated in Table 3.1,Chinese criteria related to identification and control of endemic fluorosis are being continuously improved.

Table 3.1 The national and professional health standards

Number	Name and publication number
1	Division of regions of endemic fluorosis GB 17018-2011
2	Control of areas of endemic fluorosis GB 17017-2010
3	The fluoride content of brick tea GB 19965-2005
4	Diagnosis of dental fluorosis WS/T 208-2011
5	Diagnostic criteria for endemic skeletal fluorosis WS 192-2008
6	The normal concentration of urinary fluoride in a population WS/T 256-2005
7	Determination of fluoride in the serum—The ion-selective electrode procedure WS/T 212-2001
8	Criteria for evaluation of the effects of improvements in the water supply and defluoridation measures WS/T 90-1996 (in revision)
9	Evaluation of the effectiveness of reducing fluoride intake by improving kitchen-ranges WS/T 194-1999
10	Determination of fluoride in the urine—The ion-selective electrode procedure WS/T 89-2015
11	Method for determination of total fluoride in coal and soil: The thermal hydrolysis— ion-selective electrode procedure WS/T 88-2012
12	Average daily fluoride intake by the population WS/T 87 — 1996 (in revision)

Further Reading

1. Black GV, McKay FS. Mottled teeth: an endemic developmental imperfection of the enamel of the teeth heretofore unknown in the literature of dentistry. Dent Cosmos, 1916;58(01):129-156.

2. Fawell J, Bailey K, Chilton J, Dahi E, Fewtrell L, Magara Y. Fluoride in Drinking-Water, IWA Publishing, London: World Health Organization, 2006.

3. Gao Q, Liu YJ, Guan ZZ. Oxidative stress might be a mechanism connected with the decreased alpha 7 nicotinic receptor influenced by high-concentration of fluoride in SH-SY5Y neuroblastoma cells. Toxicol In Vitro. 2008; 22(4):837-843.

4. Guan ZZ, Xiao KQ, Zeng XY, Long YG, Cheng YH, Jiang SF, Wang YN. Changed cellular membrane lipid composition and lipid peroxidation of kidney in rats with chronic fluorosis. Arch Toxicol. 2000; 74(10):602-608.

5. Guan ZZ, Wang YN, Xiao KQ, Dai DY, Chen YH, Liu JL, Sindelar P, Dallner G. Influence of chronic fluorosis on membrane lipids in rat brain. Neurotoxicol Teratol. 1998; 20(5):537-542.

6. Guan ZZ, Yang PS, Pan S, Yu LD. An experimental study of blood biochemical diagnostic indices for chronic fluorosis. Fluoride. 1989; 3(2):112-115.

7. Lyth O. Endemic fluorosis in Kweichow, China. Lancet. 1946; 247(6390):233-237.

8. Shortt HE, McRobert GR, Barnard TW, Nayar ASM. Endemic fluorosis in the Madras Presidency. Indian J Med Res. 1937; 25:553-568.

9. Zheng B, Wu D, Wang B, Liu X, Wang M, Wang A, Xiao G, Liu P, Finkelman RB. Fluorosis caused by indoor coal combustion in China: discovery and progress. Environ Geochem Health. 2007; 29(2):103-108.

10. Wei ZD, Zhou LY, Bao RC. Endemic Food-borne Fluorosis in Guizhou, China. Fluoride. 1981; 14(2):91-93.

11. Gao YH, Sun DJ, Zhao LJ, An D, Deng JY, Yang XJ, et al. Division of endemic fluorosis areas. The State Standard of the People's Republic of China, GB17018-2011.

12. COWI. Review of practical experience with defluoridation of rural water supply programmes Part 11, 73pp. Ministry of Foreign Affairs, Danida, Copenhagen, 1998.

13. Dahi, E. Contact Precipitation for defluoridation of water. Paper presented at 22nd WEDC Conference, New Delhi,1996; September 9-13, 1996.

14. Dahi E. Small community plants for low cost defluoridation of water by contact precipitation. In; Proceedings of the 2nd International Workshop on Fluorosis and Defluoridation of Water, Nazareth, November 19-22, 1997.

15. Fink, G.J, Lindsay, F.K. Activated alumina for removing fluorides from drinking water. Industrial and Engineering, 1936; 28(9), 947-948.

16. Moges G., Zwenge F, Socher M. Preliminary investigations on the defluoridation of water using fired clay chips. African Earth Sci, 1996; 21(4), 479-482.

17. Sun DJ. Endemiology. Beijing：People's Medical Publishing Press,2011.

18. Sun DJ, Gao YH. Endemic fluorosis prevention manual. Beijing：People's Medical Publishing Press,2012.

19. An D. The picture anthology about control of endemic fluorosis caused by burning coal. Guizhou: Guizhou Science and Technology press, 2012.

Guifan Sun, Guangqian Yu, Lijun Zhao, Xin Li,
Yuanyuan Xu, Bing Li, and DianJun Sun

Abstract

Arsenicosis, also described as Blackfoot Disease, was first reported in the 1950s in Taiwan, China. In the mainland of China, endemic arsenic poisoning induced by consumption of arsenic-contaminated drinking water was first reported in 1983 in Kuitun city, Xinjiang Uygur Autonomous Region. The distribution of endemic arsenicosis has also been confirmed in Inner Mongolia Autonomous Region, Shanxi, Jilin, Ningxia, Qinghai, Anhui, Gansu, Hubei, Yunnan and Shaanxi provinces. According to the recent research by Eawag, Swiss Federal Institute of Aquatic Science and Technology, there is an estimated 19. 6 million people who are at risk of being affected by arsenic-contaminated groundwater. In addition, another type of endemic arsenic poisoning is found due to burning coal containing high levels of arsenic. Consumption of arsenic-contaminated food (mainly corns and chili peppers) dried by burning coal with high concentration of arsenic, as well as inhalation of arsenic-contaminated air are the main exposure routes of this kind of arsenicosis.

The early symptoms of endemic arsenic poisoning usually occur in the skin, characterized with pigmentation changes, hard patches (hyperkeratosis) on the palms and soles. In addition to skin alterations, endemic arsenic poisoning is reported to be associated with high risk of cancers in the lung, skin, liver, prostate, bladder and kidney. The International Agency for Research on Cancer (IARC) has classified arsenic and arsenic compounds as human carcinogens. Other adverse health effects resulting from chronic ingestion of inorganic arsenic include neurotoxicity, diabetes, cardiovascular disease and respiratory complications.

This chapter mainly introduces the latest studies of etiology and epidemiology, clinical manifestations, as well as the diagnostic standard and criteria of endemic arsenicosis in China. The government of China has made great intervention progresses including provision of arsenic-safe water and improved stoves to mitigate the damage of this public health problem. What's more, establishing an effective surveillance system including accurate water quality database and dynamic GIS mapping system using a geostatistical-based risk model, is now necessary and important not only for the forthcoming large scale screening but also for the ultimate goal of arsenic elimination.

4.1 Background of Endemic Arsenic Poisoning in China

4.1.1 Discovery of Endemic Arsenic Poisoning in China

Elevated concentrations of arsenic in groundwater have been reported in many locations all over the world during the last three decades. Consumption of this groundwater adversely affects the health of over 100 million people mostly in Asia.

Arsenicosis from drinking groundwater exposure in China was first reported in the 1950s in Taiwan province characterized by Blackfoot Disease. In the mainland of China, endemic arsenicosis caused by drinking water was first reported in 1983 in Kuitun city, Xinjiang Uygur Autonomous Region. After that, investigations have identified several aquifers in inland areas of northern China where groundwater frequently contains >10 μg/L arsenic, a current drinking water standard of China for large centralized water supply.

Up to now, in addition to Xinjiang Uygur Autonomous Region, the distribution of endemic arsenicosis has been confirmed in Inner Mongolia Autonomous Region, Shanxi, Jilin, Ningxia, Qinghai, Anhui, Gansu, Hubei, Yunnan and Shaanxi provinces. By tracing the cases of arsenicosis, more and more wells in many provinces, 18 out of 31 provinces/autonomous regions in the mainland of China, were detected with high arsenic concentration in drinking water. The distributive area of arsenicosis in China is expected to be increased as large numbers of wells have been detected having high concentrations of arsenic. Tens of millions of medium to deep wells have been drilled by farmers since the 1970's economic reforms, which results in a steady improvement of living conditions in rural China. Because these tube wells often tap into arsenic-rich aquifer, a large portion of the rural population is exposed to chronic arsenic poisoning.

In addition to drinking water type of arsenicosis, there is also a type of coal-burning arsenic poisoning caused by the dried stable foods contaminated with high concentrations of arsenic as well as inhaling high-levels of arsenic indoor air. Chronic arsenic poisoning caused by coal-burning is reported mainly in different locations in Guizhou province and Shaanxi province, where local inhabitants widely use the arsenic-rich coal for cooking, heating and drying corn and hot peppers, two kinds of local staple foods.

4.1.2　Current Situation of Exposure to Natural Arsenic and Health Effects

Since the beginning of 11th five-year plan of China economy development program, the government had invested a lot of money for the mitigation of arsenic from drinking water in areas of endemic arsenicosis. Almost all the villages where patients with arsenicosis were found were facilitated with safe drinking water. The Chinese government had set arsenic standard for large centralized drinking water supply from 0.05 mg/L to 0.01 mg/L and had established the first diagnosis standard of endemic arsenic poisoning in the world. For the coal-burning type of arsenic exposure, the prevention and mitigation activities are entirely funded by the government. These included the provision of improved stoves with chimney for each household, the advice to households not to use high arsenic coal for home heating, cooking and drying staple foods, as well as the introduction of planting rice as local staple food. So far, almost all affected households have been provided with the improved stoves.

Although progresses have been made as described above, the full magnitude and scale of arsenic poisoning problems, especially for drinking-water type, remain very much unclear in China. According to the new standard limit of arsenic in drinking water, a large-scale well sampling investigation sponsored by the government was conducted, which covered 20,517 villages in 292 counties from 16 provinces in China. About 450,000 wells were sampled and arsenic concentrations were tested by field testing with the Merck arsenic kit. Results showed that about 16% of wells contained arsenic (As) over 10 μg/L and nearly 5% over 50μg/L. More than 10,000 residents were identified with arsenicosis at various degrees of skin lesions according to the National Diagnosis Standard for Endemic Arsenicosis. What has been reported is considered only the tip of the iceberg. There is an urgent need for the government to investigate the extent of endemic chronic arsenic poisoning in China for in-depth understanding the magnitude of problems and to provide timely and effective prevention and management of this silent public health calamity.

Based on an understanding of the process that affect arsenic solubility in groundwater aquifers, a geostatistical risk model that classifies safe and unsafe areas with respect to geogenic arsenic contamination in China has developed recently. The model estimates that 19.6 million people are at risk of being affected by the consumption of arsenic-contaminated groundwater according to the arsenic standard in drinking water. Although the result must be confirmed with additional field measurement, the novel arsenic map generated with the risk model pinpoints new arsenic-affected areas and highlights the potential magnitude of the health threat in China. Currently, a test of arsenic concentration out of wells were mainly focussed on localities/villages where patients with arsenicosis had been diagnosed, which would not provide more useful information for communities to take preventive action. Moreover, such discovery of high level of arsenic in drinking water is also too late for the affected population. In fact, the test of arsenic concentration out of drinking-water wells should be carried out based on the geological formation of potential high-level arsenic areas, with technical support from the Department of Geology in the provinces/autonomous Region in collaboration with the Ministry of Geology and do NOT begin just when the patients with arsenicosis have been diagnosed.

Large scale screening of arsenic concentration in the existing wells (well to well) should be planned and implemented in collaboration with the Department of Geology and the Ministry of Geology in each affected province according to the geological formation of the areas where the shallow and medium deep aquifers would most likely have naturally occurring arsenic.

Establishing an effective water quality arsenic database and GIS mapping system for long term and sustainable surveillance of arsenic in drinking water as a measure for early detection for prevention are required. Such surveillance systemcan help identify wells with high level of arsenic and other harmful elements and map out its localities in the affected villages/counties for priority action. The application of these databases and GIS mapping can display the distribution of high-level arsenic well locations, number of users of the high arsenic wells, as well as population at risk and patients with arsenicosis in villages, counties and provinces. Such surveillance system, database and GIS maps when established and utilized can be used as advocacy tools to government policy-makers for their commitment on mitigation of drinking water arsenic problems, and as effective education tools to project officers and ordinary people for guidance of early detection and planning actions on priority basis in high arsenic localities.

4.2 The Classification and Geological Environment of Endemic Arsenicosis Areas

4.2.1 Classification of Endemic Arsenic Poisoning

Endemic arsenic poisoning is classified into two types including drinking water type and coal-burning type. The former is induced by the consumption of arsenic-contaminated drinking water, whereas the latter is due to the use of coal which is the arsenic-rich fuel for cooking, heating or drying food.

4.2.1.1 Drinking Water Type

Long period of ingestion of groundwater contaminated by high level of arsenic will induce endemic arsenic poisoning of drinking water type. In China, an area with arsenic level of the groundwater beyond 0.05mg/L as well as patients with arsenicosis is defined as epidemic area of drinking water type of endemic arsenic poisoning. The area only with arsenic level of the groundwater beyond 0.05mg/L is defined as potential epidemic area. The main exposure of it is through the consumption of arsenic-contaminated drinking water extracted from pump wells (Fig. 4.1).

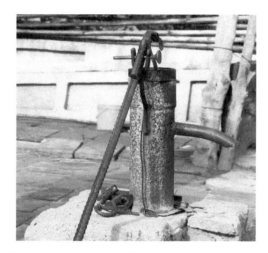

Fig. 4.1　Hand pump well with arsenic contaminated water.

Excessive exposure to arsenic through drinking water has been reported to be associated with increased prevalence of human cancers of the skin and other internal organs including lung, urinary bladder, kidney, and liver. Increasing evidence has also suggested a possible role of prolonged arsenic exposure through drinking water in the development of arsenic-induced chronic non-cancer diseases, among which hypertension and diabetes are foci of the concern. Among the arsenic-related health effects, skin lesions, including hyperpigmentation, depigmentation and hyperkeratosis are the most prominent and therefore observationally distinguishable.

4. 2. 1. 2　Coal-burning Type

Coal-burning type of endemic arsenic poisoning is unique and only found in China throughout the world. Since coal is plentiful in the epidemic areas at the surface, burning coal has become the primary fuel source for domestic use, such as cooking, heating and drying of crops and hot peppers (Fig. 4.2). According to the surveillance data of the local department of health, arsenic concentration in the coal of these areas is in the range of 417.7-2166.7 mg/kg. Routes of exposure to arsenic by burning coal is complicated, as people may be exposed through the ingestion of arsenic-contaminated foods (corns and chili peppers) which are dried by burning coal rich in arsenic, as well as through the inhalation of arsenic-contaminated air when burning coal for cooking, heating or drying food. It has been reported that arsenic concentration in the indoor air is between 0.093-0.261 mg/m^3 during the period of the domestic use of coal, and that arsenic concentration in the food dried by burning coal is in the region of 41.3-693.0 mg/kg, which is 5.9-990.0 times than that of the national standard of China. It has been estimated that 3-20mg of arsenic will be taken into the body of the individual everyday through the respiratory and digestive tract, which is from several to ten times more than the everyday intake of individual exposed to arsenic through the consumption of arsenic-contaminated drinking water.

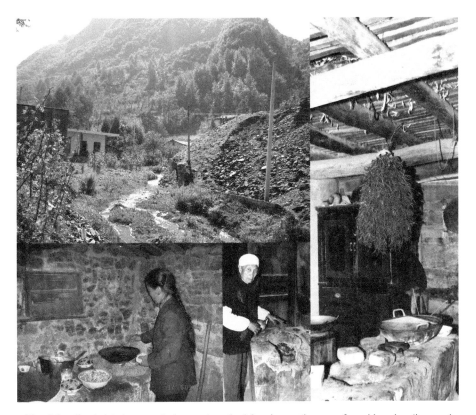

Fig. 4.2　Coal rich in arsenic is used as fuel for domestic use of cooking, heating and drying of corns and hot peppers.

Epidemic area of coal-burning type is defined as arsenic concentration in the coal beyond 100mg/kg, increase of arsenic level in the air, food and drinking water, and prevalence of endemic arsenic poisoning. Chronic exposure to high level of arsenic through burning coal in domestic living is associated with skin lesions and cancer. Patients usually die of cancers of skin, lung, breast and liver, and ascites due to cirrhosis.

4.2.2 Geological Environment of Endemic Arsenicosis Areas

Over the last decade, a large number of investigations have been carried out to delineate the spatial distribution and to characterize the chemical compositions of high-level arsenic groundwater with a focus on several inland basins in north China. Findings from these studies, including improved understanding of the hydrogeological and geochemical factors resulting in their enrichments, have been applied to guide development of clean and safe groundwater in these areas of the endemic disease.

The researches on geological environment of high-level arsenic groundwater were in several inland basins of north China including Yinchuan, Hetao and Songnen Plains, and Huhhot and Datong Basins where most endemic arsenicosis areas located. Fig. 4.3 shows the natural landscape of Huhhot Basin in Inner Mongolia. For these arid and semi-arid inland basins of north China, high-level arsenic groundwater occurs frequently in aquifers with organic-rich fluvial-lacustrine deposits, where the flat, low-lying topography leads to long residence time of groundwater that evolves to be weakly alkaline and frequently strongly reducing. Sediment arsenic concentrations are often elevated (>10mg/kg) in sands where high-level arsenic groundwater occurs.

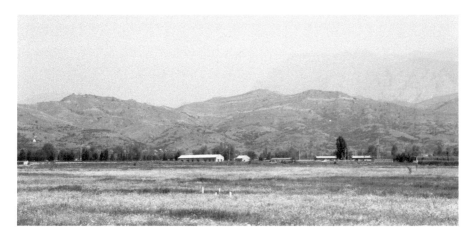

Fig. 4.3   Natural landscape of drinking water type of endemic arsenicosis areas in Huhhot Basin in Inner Mongolia. (Picture is from Prof. Xia Yajuan)

It has been known that two hydrogeological conditions favor accumulation of aqueous arsenic that is mobilized from aquifer sediment. First, the aquifer consists of sediment, which is typically geologically young and the syndepositional arsenic has not been flushed out. Second, groundwater has a long residence time due to sluggish flow in flat areas such as deltas or flood plains. This is the case for inland basins in north China as in Bangladash where the center of the basins is usually topographically low and flat, with regional groundwater flow converging from the surrounding high terrains. This convergence of flow to topographic low results in discharge through evapotranspiration and may cause further enrichment of arsenic in shallow groundwater.

Hydrochemical analysis showed that weakly alkaline to alkaline pH conditions are common for the high-level arsenic groundwater in inland basins of north China, suggesting enhanced mobility of arsenic because adsorption of arsenic to the iron minerals that are carrier phases is poor under alkaline pH conditions. Bicarbonate (HCO_3) is typically the most abundant anion, with some waters being Cl dominant. In all the basins, groundwaters evolve from Ca-dominant to Na-dominant and sometimes Cl-rich when evaporation plays a role in the low-lying parts of the basins.

In addition to the inland basins, Huaihe River Plain also has several clusters of groundwater arsenic occurrence identified through arsenic screening efforts. The Huaihe River Basin has an area of 330,000 km^2 and encompasses five provinces: Henan, Anhui, Jiangsu, Shandong and Hubei. The Basin has abundant coal deposits. The Huaihe River, the abandoned paleo-Yellow River and the Yangtze River contribute to deposition of fluvial and deltaic aquifers.

4.3 Epidemiology of Endemic Arsenic Poisoning in China

Endemic arsenic poisoning is induced by the excessive exposure to arsenic through environment. The main source of human environmental exposure is through consumption of drinking water contaminated by arsenic. Populations at risk of exposure to excessive levels of arsenic through drinking water have been emerging since the 1960s. Up to now, arsenic-contaminated drinking water has been a major problem in public health of China. According to the recent research of Eawag, Swiss Federal Institute of Aquatic Science and Technology, there is an estimated 19.6 million people who are at risk of being affected by the consumption of arsenic-contaminated groundwater.

In addition to arsenicosis induced by the consumption of arsenic-contaminated drinking water, there is another type of endemic arsenic poisoning which is due to burning coal containing high levels of arsenic. Consumption of arsenic-contaminated food (corns and chili peppers) which are dried by burning coal with high concentration of arsenic, as well as inhalation of arsenic-contaminated air are the main exposure routes of this kind of arsenicosis. It is the unique poisoning induced by arsenic which was only found in China throughout the world.

4.3.1　Geographic Distribution

Endemic arsenic poisoning of drinking water type was first identified in southwest Taiwan in the 1950s, where a strange epidemic dermatosis which was known as black foot disease latter was discovered. The epidemic region covered 56 towns, 7 cities and counties in the north of Taiwan and Jiayi area. In the mainland of China, the first epidemic area was found in Xinjiang province in the west part of China in 1983. After that, a few provinces had performed clue investigations about the endemic arsenicosis caused by intake of high arsenic in drinking water. From the beginning of 1980s to the end of the twentieth century, it was successively confirmed that endemic arsenicosis had been distributed in Inner Mongolia, Xinjiang, Shanxi, Jilin, and Ningxia, by measuring the content of arsenic in drinking water and inspecting the lesion of skin.

Since 2000, to analyze the distribution of arsenic levels in drinking water comprehensively in Chinese mainland, the Chinese government had used funding supports from the Central Finance and UNICEF and had organized a comprehensive screening of drinking water sources with high levels of arsenic. Merck semi-quantitative arsenic kit was applied in the field testing financed by the UNICEF. A total of 36,820 villages in 18 provincial areas were investigated, and over 3.6 million water samples were measured. The investigation has been the most comprehensive study of water sources with high levels of arsenic in China so far. It is also the most comprehensive and the largest-scale investigation on high-arsenic area distribution in the world. Any possible areas with high-arsenic levels in drinking water were investigated, which basically clarified the geographic distribution of high-arsenic levels in drinking water and the threatened population. According to the national standards for arsenic levels of less than 50 µg/L arsenic for small-scale centralized water supply and non-centralized water supply among household tube wells, 1,894,587 inhabitants out of 2,476 villages were identified at risk of exposure to high levels of arsenic, including 32,673,677 inhabitants in all the 36,820 villages. However, according to the national standard requiring arsenic levels of less than 10 µg/L for large-scale centralized water supply and related standards of World Health Organization (WHO), 6,095,316 inhabitants were at risk of exposure to high levels of arsenic. The result of the survey represented the most comprehensive distribution of arsenic levels in drinking water in China. Eventually, high-arsenic areas were distributed in 18 provinces and autonomous regions including Inner Mongolia, Shanxi, Anhui, Qinghai, Ningxia, Xinjiang, Gansu, Jilin, Jiangsu, Shaanxi, Hubei, Hunan, Jiangxi, Henan, Shandong, Heilongjiang, Yunnan, and Sichuan (Table 4.1).

Table 4.1 Distribution of high arsenic areas in China mainland and the coverage of population

Province	As> 10 µg/L			As> 50 µg/L		
	Counties (n)	Villages (n)	Population (thousand)	Counties (n)	Villages (n)	Population (thousand)
Anhui	23	266	541	16	99	198
Gansu	16	162	185	9	44	46
Henan	46	299	412	6	30	44
Heilongjiang	11	30	24	3	6	5
Hubei	22	413	647	17	189	294
Hunan	1	13	1	1	6	1
Jilin	11	947	510	7	301	135
Jiangsu	7	81	151	5	35	66
Jiangxi	8	28	34	5	9	11
Inner Mongolia	51	1904	683	34	925	357

Continue

Province	As> 10 µg/L			As> 50 µg/L		
	Counties (n)	Villages (n)	Population (thousand)	Counties (n)	Villages (n)	Population (thousand)
Ningxia	6	140	62	6	80	37
Qinghai	19	83	57	7	28	17
Shandong	46	264	364	18	46	82
Shanxi	29	619	847	17	156	204
Shannxi	28	114	129	5	14	17
Sichuan	7	134	27	4	55	10
Xinjiang	100	1528	1291	50	397	310
Yunnan	20	138	132	16	56	61
Total	451	7163	6095	226	2476	1895

Recently, a research group from Eawag, Swiss Federal Institute of Aquatic Science and Technology published their findings in *Science*. According to this paper, there is an estimated 19.6 million people are at risk of being affected by the consumption of arsenic-contaminated groundwater. Findings of this research is based on a statistical risk model that classifies safe and unsafe areas with respect to geogenic arsenic contamination in China, using the threshold of 0.01 mg/L, the World Health Organization guideline and current Chinese standard for drinking water. The model forecasts that the area at risk of groundwater arsenic contamination (>0.01 mg/L) may encompass more than 580,000 km², and it pinpoints elevated arsenic concentrations in regions where endemic arsenic poisoning has already been detected. Large areas such as Tarim basin (Xinjiang), Ejina basin (Inner Mongolia), Heihe basin (Gansu), Qaidam basin (Qinghai), the Northeastern plain (Inner Mongolia, Jilin, and Liaoning), and the North China plain (Henan and Shandong) were identified as being potentially affected. Although the results must be confirmed with additional field measurements, this risk model identifies numerous arsenic-affected areas and highlights the potential magnitude of this health threat in China.

Coal-burning type of endemic arsenic poisoning only exist in China throughout the world. Patients of this kind of poisoning were firstly identified in Guizhou

Province, southwest region of China, in 1970s. This area was designated as epidemic area of coal-burning type of endemic arsenic poisoning in the 1990s. According to a report of 2002, approximately 70,000-200,000 residents in Xingren, Xingyi, Anlong, Zhijin, Kaiyang and Jinhua counties of Guizhou Province were at risk of exposure to high levels of arsenic. Later reports by the Guizhou Center for Disease Control and prevention of 2005 indicated that more than 2,800 patients were identified in the Xingren, Xingyi, Anlong and Zhijin counties. The south part of Shanxi province was subsequently designated as another epidemic area of coal-burning type poisoning with a shorter history than that of Guizhou province.

4.3.2 Population Distribution

Large quantities of evidences from epidemiological investigations indicated that individuals will suffer from endemic arsenic poisoning at any age if being exposed to arsenic at high concentration and accumulated too much arsenic in the body through drinking water or burning coal. The youngest patient of drinking water type poisoning is only 6-month-old who was found in a village of Shanxi province. Incidence of poisoning in the group of old people is more severe than that in the group of young people. The peak age suffer from poisoning is found to be between 40 and 50 years old. Young patients, mainly among primary and middle school students, will occur in the regions contaminated by extremely high level of arsenic.

Incidence rate of male is higher than that of female, which may be due to the high intake of arsenic-contaminated water and food in male population.

Since there is no centralized water supply system in most of the region of the rural areas, where ground water without health surveillance is the main source of drinking water, most of the cases of endemic arsenic poisoning of drinking water type are found among the residents of rural areas. Coal-burning type poisoning also occurs in the remote mountain villages of rural area where the traditional habit of drying food by open furnace is still in use.

Since family members are usually exposed to the same level of arsenic through drinking water or burning coal, cases of endemic arsenic poisoning seem to be clustered with in families. More than two members of the same family suffer from poisoning is a usual phenomenon in the epidemic areas. In some families, all members are found to be patients of endemic arsenic poisoning.

Some enzymes involved the process of arsenic metabolism have gene polymorphisms, such as GSTO1 and GSTO2 from glutathione-S-transferase (GST) family and arsenic 3-methyltransferase (AS3MT), all of which play an important role in the methylation metabolism of arsenic in the liver. It has been indicated that gene polymorphism of these enzymes is associated with the different susceptibilities among individuals living in the same exposure environment.

4.4 Mechanism of arsenicosis

The mechanism underlying arsenic toxicity has been fully elucidated. Arsenic is mainly existed with inorganic forms in the natural world and is biomethylated into monomethylated and dimethylated forms in humans. Inorganic arsenic and its metabolites are different in toxicity but similar in mode of action. In vivo and in vitro studies suggest these arsenicals can induce gene deletion, chromosomal alterations (aberrations, aneuploidy, and sister chromatid exchanges), comutagenicity, oxidative stress, cell proliferation and inhibition of mitochondrial respiration. Recent studies also provide compelling evidence that arsenic targets stem cells for the development of various diseases including cancer, developmental abnormalities, as well as many other disorders. In addition, epigenetic alterations such as cytosine DNA methylation at CpG sites, covalent post-translational histone modifications, and microRNAs, are indicated in arsenic toxicity, particularly due to long-term health effects from prenatal arsenic exposure.

4.5 Clinical Manifestations

The early symptoms of endemic arsenic poisoning usually occur in the skin, characterized with pigmentation changes, hard patches (hyperkeratosis) on the palms and soles. In addition to skin alterations, chronic exposure to arsenic may cause cancers of various organs in humans. The International Agency for Research on Cancer (IARC) has classified arsenic and arsenic compounds as human carcinogens. Endemic arsenic poisoning is reported to be associated with high risk of cancers in the lung, skin, liver, prostate, bladder and kidney. Other adverse health effects resulting from chronic ingestion of inorganic arsenic include neurotoxicity, diabetes, cardiovascular disease and respiratory complications.

The duration of arsenic exposure with the date of onset of symptoms does not follow a particular time frame. In Xinjiang Province of China, typical skin lesions were found in patients after three years of arsenic exposure. Skin lesions have been reported to occur after drinking arsenic contaminated water for one year or even less in West Bengal. In Taiwan, China, the youngest patient with hyper-pigmentation was 3-year-old. Among the population exposed to arsenic in drinking water in Chile, cases of cutaneous arsenicosis, including both pigmentation and hyperkeratosis, had been described in children as young as two years of age. In 1943, Rattner and Dorne reported the development of hyperpigmentation within 6-12 months after using arsenic as a medicine at a dose of 4.75 mg/day. Hyperkeratosis appeared after approximately three years. Hence a history of chronic arsenic exposure for more than six months is essential for typical skin manifestation.

4.5.1 Hyperkeratoses

Characteristic hyperkeratoses are located predominantly on the palms and soles of the feet, which are symmetrical, translucent and pale yellow or tan keratotic small non-inflammatory papules (Fig. 4.4). Verrucous hyperkeratosis presents with cauliflower-like surfaces. At the very early stage, subcutaneous mini-papules have an indurated, grit like phenotype, which can be best appreciated by palpation. The lesions usually advance to form raised, punctated, 2-4 mm wart-like keratosis which is easily visible.

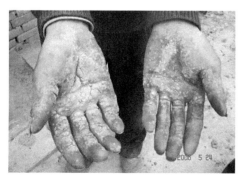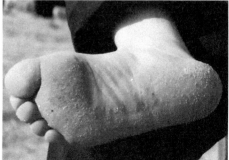

Fig. 4.4　Hyperkeratosis on palm and sole.

Later, they form small papules and verrucae and subsequently interfuse into pieces. Eventually, hyperkeratoses decrease the patients' working ability.

4. 5. 2 Hyper-pigmentation and/or Hypo-pigmentation on the Skin

Skin pigment changes usually take place in unexposed parts of the body and distribute symmetrically. An alteration of specific pigmentation depends on individual circumstances. Hyper-pigmentation is an overall body skin darkening into a grey and slight black color. The hypo-pigmentation is existed in combination with hyper-pigmentation, presenting with shapes of pin heads, rice grains or raindrops, locally known as "flower skin disease". In severe cases, even oral mucosa and the genitals can be affected (Fig. 4.5).

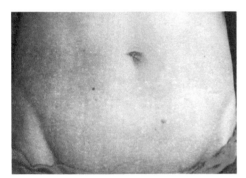

Fig. 4.5   Skin hyper-pigmentation and hypo-pigmentation on the trunk.

4. 5. 3 Bowen's Disease and Skin Cancer

Keratosis areas on the palms and soles, or spotted melanosis on the body, may deteriorate and lead to surface roughness, erosion, ulceration, pain and surrounding skin flush, and finally result in Bowen's disease or skin cancer (Fig. 4.6). This process can take as long as 30-40 years. Bowen's disease shows up in single or multiple sites in the skin. Skin cancer is relatively distinctive in endemic arsenic poisoning. The lesions are frequently multiple and involve unexposed areas of the body, contrary to non-arsenical skin cancer which usually presents as a single lesion occurs in exposed parts of the body. Pathological diagnosis for Bowen's disease and skin cancer only can be made by biopsy.

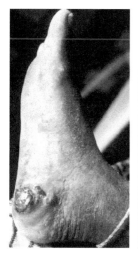 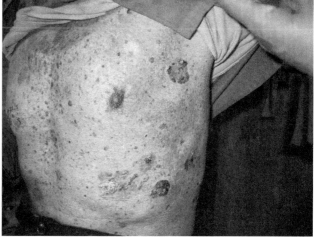

Fig. 4.6   Arsenic hyperkeratosis and pigmentation plaque could develop into basal cell carcinoma (left) and Bowen's disease (right), one kinds of skin cancer

4. 5. 4   Histopathology of Skin Lesions

Histopathology of epidermis shows active hyperplasia, deformed structure and thick layers of basal cells, spinous cells and cuticles (Fig. 4.8). Leathery base of the heightened dermal layer causes sponge-like performance without loss of basement membrane integrity. Keratinocytes are often filled with blue stained alkalophilic particles with disappearance of condensation nuclei and denuclearization. Spinous cells are different in size and shape, showing vacuoles and red staining keratosis capsules. Megakaryocytes, multinucleated giant cells can also be seen in these two kinds of cells. Sometimes there is an infiltration of small round cells, edema, thickening of subcutaneous small arterial wall, and proliferation of glial fiber in the dermal layer.

Involvement of the dorsum of the extremities and the trunk in arsenic hyperkeratoses has also been reported. Trunk and dorsum with hyperkeratoses show rash areas in brown or black. Keratoses are slightly raised, varying in size and rough in texture. Some of the lesions show dark red erosion on surface. Histopathologically, there is often horny thickening, epidermal hyperplasia at different cell layers and decreased depth of skin papillae. Papillae may become widened and penetrate the dermal layer. Normal structure of basal cell and spinous cell layers becomes chaotic and deformed. Spinous cells frequently degenerated. Basal cells and whip cells show a lot of brown particles. Nuclei of these cells show enhanced splitting and give rise to multinucleated cells. Keratosis occurs with individual cells, and sometimes larger keratosis capsule full of red staining keratin are prominent.

Some patients develop basal-cell carcinoma or squamous cell carcinoma, with loss of normal skin structure and dermal infiltration by the cancerous tissue (Fig.4.7). Some keratotic areas are histopathologically similar to senile keratoses or appear flat like ringworm, psoriasis and other skin conditions.

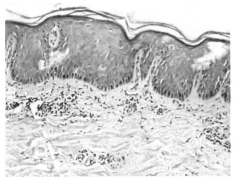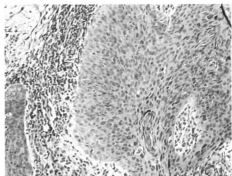

Fig. 4.7   Histopathology of Skin Lesions: Obvious cell hyperplasia at the stratum spinosum, chronic infiltration of new inflammatory cells at the shallow layer of dermis, and hyper-pigmentation at the staratum basale (HE stain, Low magnification) (left); Canceration throughout the epidermis, and being Bowen's disease of skin (right). (Pictures are from Prof.Aihua Zhang)

4. 5. 5   Other Cancers and Non-Cancer Manifestations

Though other types of cancers, e.g. lung cancer, bladder cancer, kidney cancer, prostate cancer, angiosarcoma of the liver are observed in significantly high number among cases of endemic arsenicosis, these have no typical characteristics suggestive of arsenic etiology. Though the various non-cancer manifestations occur in association with endemic arsenicosis, nothing is specific except for skin manifestations.

(1) Nervous system: Effect of arsenic poisoning on central nervous system causes severe headache, dizziness, memory impairment, and vision and/or hearing loss. Effect on peripheral nerve is related to progressive numbness, glove and/or

stocking paresthesias, and decreased sensory nerve conduction. Impairment of neurodevelopment in children is also reported by many epidemiological studies, in which a dose-response relationship between cognitive function and arsenic concentrations in tap water or toenail has been observed.

(2) Digestive system: Symptoms of digestive system include dyspepsia, loss of appetite, nausea, abdominal pain and diarrhea. Hepatomegaly or cirrhosis may also develop.

(3) Circulatory system: Peripheral vascular disorders are common in endemic arsenic poisoning areas. Many people complain of cold intolerance. Raynaud's disease is often seen. In Province of Taiwan, China, arsenic exposure has been linked to "Blackfoot Disease", which is a severe disease of blood vessels leading to gangrene. However, this disease has not been observed in other parts of the world, and it is possible that malnutrition contributes to its development. In addition, population studies relate an increased incidence of ischemic heart disease, hypertension and cardiovascular mortality with chronic exposure to high levels of arsenic.

(4) Respiratory system: Difficulty breathing, wheezing and cough may appear. Chronic bronchitis with or without obstruction are the common cause of mortality in many cases of chronic arsenic toxicity. So, it is extremely important that bronchial irritation should be reduced to a minimum.

(5) Endocrine system: Endemic arsenic poisoning is suggested to induce type 2 diabetic mellitus through interfering with insulin-stimulated signal transduction pathway or with critical steps in glucose metabolism.

4.6 Diagnostic Criteria of Endemic Arsenicosis in China

4.6.1 Diagnosis Indexes

4.6.1.1 Essential Indexes

The resident living in the endemic arsenicosis area having exposure to excessive high arsenic and showing one of following manifestations can be diagnosed as the patient with endemic arsenicosis. (1) Papule-like, nodule-like, or wart-like hyperkerotosis on palms and soles, the cause of which is difficult to elucidate. (2) Diffuse or sporadic hyper-pigmentation spots and/or circle hypo-pigmentation spots with hazy border in different sizes from millet to soya bean on the un-exposed skin of trunk, the cause of which is difficult to elucidate.

4.6.1.2 *Referential Indexes*

Arsenic content of resident urine or hair sample in endemic areas is significantly higher than that of resident urine or hair sample in non-endemic areas.

4.6.2 Dermatological Metamorphosis Classifications

4.6.2.1 *Hyperkeratosis on Palms and Soles*

Grade I: There are three or more sporadic papule-like or nodule-like hyperkeratosis showing the size of rice on palms and soles that can be seen by visual inspection and/ or by touching.

Grade II: There are more or larger obvious papule-like hyperkeratosis on palms and soles.

Grade III: There is extensive hyperkeratosis in different shapes of plaque or streak on the palms and soles, and multiple and bigger wart-like hyperkeratosis simultaneously on the palms and soles, and on the back of the hands and feet, which chap and become ulcer with bleeding on the surface.

4.6.2.2 *Cutaneous Hyper-pigmentation*

Grade I: Slightly darker pigment of the skin of the un-exposed body, mainly on the trunk, or the sporadic symmetrical light brown hyper-pigmentation spots on the skin.

Grade II: Skin pigment, mainly on the un-exposed trunk, becomes gray, or the appearance of many brown hyper-pigmentation spots in different shades on the skin.

Grade III: Skin pigment, mainly on the un-exposed trunk, becomes dark gray, or the appearance of extensive and intensive brown hyper-pigmentation spots, or lots of dark brown or black hyper-pigmentation plaques having diameter of 1 cm on the skin.

4.6.2.3 *Cutaneous Hypo-pigmentation*

Grade I: The appearance of symmetric and sporadic hypo-pigmentation spots in size of pinpoint on the un-exposed skin, mainly on the trunk.

Grade II:The appearance of more spotted hypo-pigmentation with hazy border on the un-exposed skin, mainly on the trunk.

Grade III:The appearance of extensive and intensive spotted hypo-pigmentation with hazy border on the un-exposed skin, mainly on the trunk.

4.6.2.4　Bowen's Disease and Skin Cancer

Hyperkeratosis areas on the palms and soles result in erosion, ulcer and pain; hyperkeratosis or pigmentation plaque on the trunk becomes dark and results in crude surface, erosion, ulcer, pain, and surrounding skin flush. The diagnosis should be confirmed by pathological biopsy.

4.6.3　Classification of Clinical Diagnosis

4.6.3.1　Suspicious Cases (With One of the Following Symptoms)

The presence of Grade I hyper-pigmentation or Grade I hypo-pigmentation, or the appearance of only have one to two papule-like or nodule-like hyperkeratosis having the size of rice on the palms and soles. Inhabitants living in the coal-burning endemic areas would develop significant visual deterioration, hypogeusia, and poor appetite.

4.6.3.2　Mild Cases (With One of the Following Symptoms)

Presence of Grade I hyperkeratosis on the palms and soles, or simultaneous appearance of Grade I hyper-pigmentation and Grade I hypo-pigmentation on the skin of trunk. Arsenic levels in urine and hair samples of the suspicious patients are obviously higher than that the normal level found in the non-endemic areas of the same region.

4.6.3.3　Moderate Cases

One of the symptoms of hyperkeratosis on the palms and soles, hyper-pigmentation and hypo-pigmentation on the skin of trunk is in Grade II degree.

4.6.3.4　Severe Cases

One of the symptoms of hyperkeratosis on the palms and soles, hyper-pigmentation and hypo-pigmentation on the skin of trunk is in Grade II degree.

4.6.3.5　Bowen's Disease and Skin Cancer

To be confirmed by pathological biopsy.

4.6.4 Skin Lesions as the Major Diagnosis Index

Clinical investigations indicate that chronic arsenic poisoning induces harmful effects to various organs in the human body, including injury of the nervous system and peripheral circulation disturbance. The resultant skin lesions are most prominent and therefore observationally distinguishable. Also, skin lesions induced by arsenicosis tend to emerge at a relative early stage and are of such specificity that they make for easy examination and diagnosis. Thus, guidelines for diagnosis of arsenicosis are basedmainly upon symptoms of skin lesion manifestation (as shown in 4.6.2 Dermatological metamorphosis classifications).

4.7 Definition and Classification of Endemic Arsenicosis Area

4.7.1 The Definition of Endemic Arsenicosis Area

Based on standards and definition of endemic arsenicosis in China, three factors must be satisfied to define the endemic area of arsenicosis. First, arsenic level in drinking water is over 0.05 mg/L, excluding man-made pollution, and in the burning coal areas, residents using the coal in open stoves have arsenic level higher than 40 mg/kg. Second, patients with endemic arsenicosis are diagnosed based on the specific skin symptoms. Third, patients' symptoms of the endemic arsenicosis are caused by consuming high arsenic drinking water, eating arsenic contaminated foods and breathing high arsenic air, and not by other arsenic sources and other diseases.

4.7.2 Classification of Endemic Arsenicosis Area

There are two types of endemic arsenicosis areas in china, namely drinking water type caused by drinking arsenic contaminated ground water and coal-burning type caused by burning high arsenic coal in the open stove in the household. The severity of the endemic area is classified according to the arsenic level in water or coal together with the prevalence rate of inhabitants' arsenicosis, and the arsenic level in water or coal is given top priority prior to the prevalence when inconsistency exists.

4. 7. 2. 1   Drinking Water Type of Endemic Arsenicosis Area

Potential endemic arsenicosis area, where the arsenic level in drinking water is more than 0.05mg/L but no arsenicosis patient is diagnosed.

Mild endemic arsenicosis area, where the arsenic level in drinking water is more than 0.10 mg/L and the prevalence rate of arsenicosis is less than 10%.

Moderate endemic arsenicosis area, where the arsenic level in drinking water is over 0.30 mg/L and the prevalence rate of arsenicosis is between 10% and 30%.

Severe endemic arsenicosis area, where the arsenic level in drinking water is higher than 0.50 mg/L, and the prevalence rate of arsenicosis is more than 30% with patients manifesting severe arsenicosis symptoms.

4. 7. 2. 2   Coal-burning Type of Endemic Arsenicosis Area

Potential endemic arsenicosis area, where the arsenic level in coal is more than 40.0 mg/kg but no arsenicosis patient is diagnosed.

Mild endemic arsenicosis area, where the arsenic level in coal is more than 100. 0 mg/kg and the prevalence rate of arsenicosis is less than 10%.

Moderate endemic arsenicosis area, where the arsenic level in coal is over 200.0 mg/kg and the prevalence rate of arsenicosis is between 10% and 30%.

Severe endemic arsenicosis area, where the arsenic level in coal is higher than 400 mg/kg, and the prevalence rate of arsenicosis is more than 30% with patients manifesting severe arsenicosis symptoms.

4.8   China's Approach for Prevention and Control of endemic arsenicosis

The government's procedures to prevent endemic arsenicosis in China include five steps: early detection of arsenic contamination in drinking water, foods and environment as well as diagnosis of patients with arsenicosis; development of guideline and criteria for the practice of prevention and control; provision of arsenic-safe water and improvement of the open stoves; surveillance; and health education.

4. 8. 1 Early Detection and Prevention

For effective dealing with the emerging chronic arsenic poisoning problem in China, the government is coordinating with various agencies to test arsenic concentration of wells in affected areas and to identify patients with arsenicosis. The former Ministry of Health, with the support of local provincial governments, is responsible for testing the arsenic concentration of wells in the affected areas. Also, UNICEF has provided some financial assistance in carrying out wide-scale testing of arsenic concentration of wells in high-risk areas. A practical method of sampling 10 percent of wells in affected areas (using village as a unit) where water samples are taken from wells in five locations (east, south, west, north and centre) has been developed based on the accumulated field experience. This method is to determine whether wide-scale testing of arsenic contents of all wells in a particular village is necessary. When one well in 10 percent surveyed has an arsenic level higher than the government standard of 0.05 mg/L, all wells in the village are then tested. The wells having arsenic levels higher than 0. 05 mg/L are marked and mapped, indicating the range of arsenic concentration. This type of mapping serves as an effective motivational tool to advise people to use their neighbors' wells that are arsenic-safe as an interim measure while waiting for the provision of an arsenic-safe water supply. National and provincial databases of high arsenic and arsenicosis villages have been developed based on the available data. These databases become a valuable tool to advocate the government for allocation of funds and for the provision of arsenic-safe water supplies to the affected rural population, with priority given to the areas having the highest arsenic level in wells.

4. 8. 2 Guideline and Criteria Related to Endemic Arsenicosis

Following detection of endemic arsenicosis in extensive area in China, Chinese specialists in arsenic research, clinicians, epidemiologists and toxicologists had developed some national or professional guideline and criteria for the prevention and control of endemic arsenecosis. The list of these criteria is shown in Table 4.2. These criteria have proven to be an important tool and reference guideline in the practice.

Table 4.2　The guideline and criteria related to Endemic arsenicosis

Number	Name and publication number
1	Tentative guideline for the classification of endemic arsenism area and clinical diagnosis 1994 (abandoned)
2	Diagnosis of endemic arsenicosis WS/T 211-2001/2015
3	Definition and division standard for endemic arsenism WS 277-2007/under revision
4	Elimination of the endemic arsenism areas GB 28595-2012
5	Determination of arsenic in urine by hydride generation atomic fluorescence spectrometry WS/T 474-2015

4. 8. 3　Provision of Arsenic-safe Water and Improved Stoves

The fundamental measure to control water-drinking type endemic arsenicosis is to cut off arsenic-rich water source. Two measures were adopted for the prevention of water-drinking type endemic arsenicosis in China. The main preventive measure is to stop drinking the original arsenic-rich water, and to construct centralized water supply system for providing alternative qualified arsenic-safe water, which included drilling a new well with arsenic-free water, changing to use the neighbour's well with low arsenic, bringing water from the river, lake and spring, building a water cellar for collecting rains, mixing the arsenic-rich water with arsenic-free water, and so on. Among them, the extensive prevention measure is to construct the water supply project and to utilize groundwater and surface water in China (Fig.4.8). The Ministry of Water Resources is working with local governments to provide arsenic-safe piped water supplies in accordance with the recommendations of the former Ministry of Health. Lots of prevention practices have verified that these projects can be used for long time and is convenient for maintenance and management as well as can get good preventive effect. When a new water supply project is built, however, it must be cautious in the selection of arsenic-safe water sources based on the data of hydrogeology. For ensuring the arsenic concentration of the new project being consistent with the national drinking water standard, the water quality must be tested while starting and completing of the water supply project. And the water should be monitored regularly during application to avoid arsenic to be increased again in drinking water.

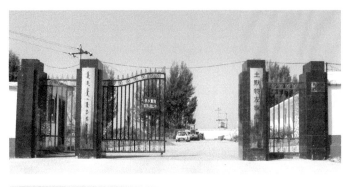

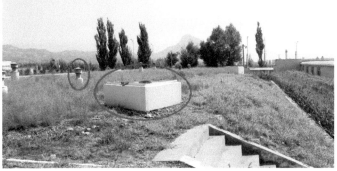

Fig. 4.8 Water works named Cilao in Tumoterzuoqi in Inner Mongolia Autonomous Region. This water works has 4 electromechanical wells and 96.23 km pipe network, covering 98 km^2 and providing arsenic-safe water for a population of 44.5 million. The original highest level of water arsenic in this endemic area is as high as 1.86mg/L; Upper: The gate of the water works; Middle: Cistern of the water works. The small oval indicates air vent hole and the big oval indicates entrance of the cistern; Lower: The distribution map of pipe network of the water works. (Pictures are from Prof. Yajuan Xia)

In addition to switching to alternative water source, another measure is to remove excessive arsenic from drinking water by utilizing physical or chemical methods in the region of no arsenic-safe water source available, so that arsenic content in drinking water can meet the national standard. These methods include coagulation, direct precipitation, ion-interchange membrane separation, bio-treatment, and so on. Generally speaking, facilities for removing arsenic from drinking water are complicated for operation and more cost, which cannot be afford by common people living in rural or poor regions far away. The effect of these facilities is not perfect in the practical prevention. In fact, these methods are rarely used in the steppe or mountain areas, where people inhabit sparsely and it is unsuitable for them to build a centralized water supply project. Millions of villagers in Bangladesh are exposed to high level of arsenic from drinking well-water. Some measures are adopted to reduce arsenic exposure in this country, such as arsenic contaminated well water painting or mapping and using arsenic removing equipments (Fig. 4.9). Limitations of using arsenic removing equipments in Bangladesh are most the same as that in China.

In coal-burning arsenic affected areas, an improved stove was mainly adopted for controlling of arsenicosis, which means to abandon the original opening stove and provide the improved stove with chimney to the affected households for venting away the smoke from the house so that the pollution of harmful material such as arsenic was decreased effectively. Resultantly, the indoor air quality was in accord

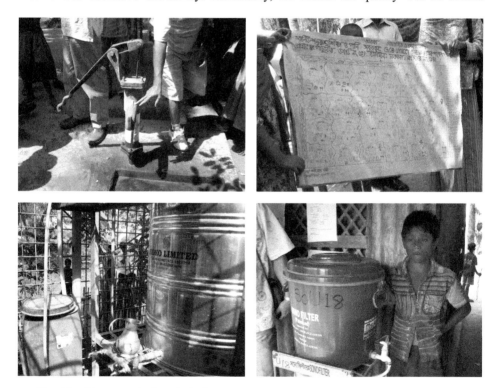

Fig. 4.9 Measures in Bangladesh to reduce arsenic exposure. Upper left: Wells with arsenic safe water are painted green, and that with arsenic contaminated are painted red. Upper right: Map of the distribution of household with arsenic contaminated water. Lower left: Equipment for removing arsenic. Lower right: Household-level filter for removing arsenic. (Pictures are from Prof. Dianjun Sun)

with the national standard for arsenic in air of residential areas. Meanwhile, habitants changed methods for food drying and keeping. The first one was to promote crops to be matured in short term by utilizing sprout cultivation under plastic film so that crops could be dried by the natural sunshine before rainy season. The second method was to dry the crops by utilizing the tobacco flue-curing barn, closed type kang or heated pipeline instead of using an opening coal-burning stove. The third method was to keep the dried food into a bag, a box or a storeroom to avoid being contaminated by arsenic-rich smoke dust. The most essential preventive measures of coal-burning type endemic arsenicosis are to prohibit mining and using arsenic-rich coal. After the mine fields with arsenic-coal were proved around the affected areas, clear energies such as sewage gas, electricity, and liquefied gas, are used to replace the source of high arsenic coal thoroughly (Fig. 4.10).

4. 8. 4 Surveillance

To investigate the prevalence of arsenicosis and the situation of control measures implemented in endemic aresenecosis area of China, a national surveillance of endemic arsenicosis has been started since 2005. The surveillance is carried out among the same spots in some affected provinces every year. The content of the surveillance includes the progress of control measures adopted in endemic areas, the prevalence of arsenicosis and urinary arsenic level of local residents, arsenic concentration in drinking water for drinking water type of endemic arsenicosis, arsenic concentration in coal, corn and hot pepper for coal-burning type of endemic arsenicosis, as well as the quality and usage of improved stoves. Resultant data of the surveillance provide the foundation of for the strategy adopted in the endemic arsenicosis control in China.

4. 8. 5 Health Education

The overall principle of endemic arsenicosis control is to stop the source of arsenic exposure as well as to decrease the intake of the arsenic. Meanwhile, health education and health promotion must be carried out among local inhabitants and officials at all levels, to increase their consciousness of controlling arsenicosis and to implement prevention measures consciously, especially for coal-burning type of endemic

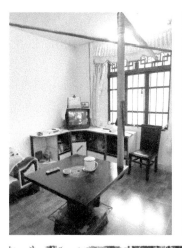
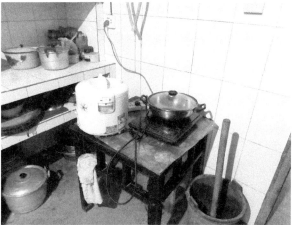
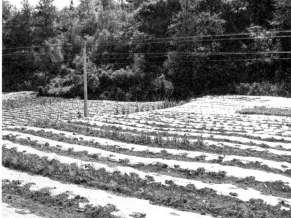
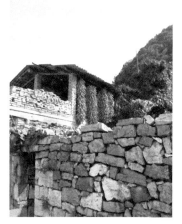

Fig. 4.10   Measures to remove arsenic in coal-burning type of endemic arsenicosis areas. Upper left: Improved stove with cover and chimney. Upper right: Rice cooker and electromagnetic oven used instead of old open stove in the families. Lower left: Film seeding in order to harvest the corn before rainy season. Lower right: Corns dried outside by sun naturally. (Pictures are from Prof. Dianjun Sun)

arsenicosis (Fig. 4.11). Then, the inhabitants can change their unhealthy behavior into healthy habit and joined in the disease control voluntarily and actively. Health education is a prime and permanent method of increasing the efficiency of preventive measures and implementing disease control sustainably.

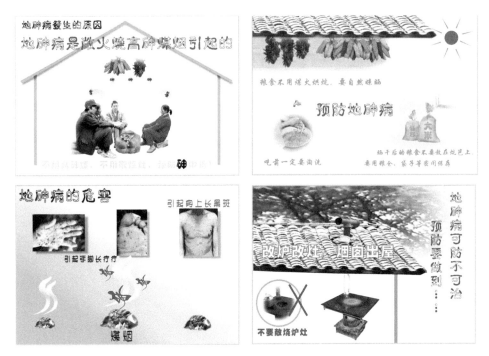

Fig. 4.11 Picture posters for health education in coal-burning type of endemic arsenicosis areas. (Pictures are from Prof. An Dong and Li Dasheng)

4.9 China's Achievement and Experience

Because endemic arsenicosis damaged residents' health severely, Chinese government has paid close attention to the mitigation and control of the disease, and has implemented preventive measures positively. By the end of 1984, the preventive measures had been implemented by provision of alternative arsenic-safe water in all the affected areas with relative higher arsenic content in drinking water in Kuitun, Xinjiang, where the arsenic affected areas was first discovered in Chinese mainland, and the preventive measures had worked effectively for the control of arsenicosis. By 2000, the alternative arsenic-safe water supply system had been implemented in all arsenic-affected areas with arsenic content in drinking water over 0.3mg/L in Inner Mongolia. Since endemic arsenicosis was managed as one of the national key endemic disease in 1992, a great effort of implementing prevention measures had been made and the progress of the disease control had achieved remarkable achievements during the past 20 years. Especially, after 2001, the implementing process of the preventive measures has been accelerated more further by enhancing investment in financial resource and manpower, and implementing the national water supply project for people and livestock, as well as implementing the national "the eleventh five-year plan" and the "the twelfth five-year plan" safe drinking water project provision in rural areas. By the end of 2012, the alterative arsenic-safe water supply systems were constructed in 93.56% arsenicosis villages, the normal operation rate was 89.13%, and the real beneficial population was 0.52 million. The water supply systems were also constructed in 1738 high arsenic villages, in which arsenic content in drinking water was over limit of national standard but no person was diagnosed as the patient with arsenicosis. The water improvement rate of those villages was 86.25%, the normal operation rate was 93.67%, and the beneficial population was 1.14 million. Nearly 90% population potentially affected by the water-arsenic was arsenicosis-free through the whole country; the severe epidemic situation has been controlled in good condition. The data from a few years surveillance began at 2009 demonstrated that after water improvement among the drinking water type endemic areas, the condition of endemic arsenicosis was relative stable, and the prevalence rate was kept at a low level. By the end of 2012, no new patient with skin cancer was found.

Coal-burning type of endemic arsenicosis only occurred in Guizhou and Shaanxi provinces in China. By employing special fund for public health provided by the central government, two provinces had implemented the control measures by stove-improving in all the arsenic-affected families during three years. Up to 2007, total 374 thousand households in 1367 coal-burning arsenic affected villages of two provinces had been provided with the improved stove, and the appropriate operation rate reached to 92.23%. All the coal-burning type of endemic arsenicosis is under control now. Just like drinking water type, the prevalence rate of arsenicosis is also kept at a relative stable level after the implementation of stove-improving. And, by 2012, no new patient with arsenicosis and skin cancer had occurred in the very severe province, Guizhou, during four-year period.

China experiences in the prevention and control of endmemic arsenicosis are summarized as follows: firstly, to organize the most comprehensive and the largest-scale investigation on high-arsenic area distribution in the world; secondly, to construct a high-quality team for disease prevention and control, especially professional institutions for the prevention and control of endemic diseases have been carrying out studies for many years on the relationship between arsenic exposure and arsenicosis; thirdly, to invest a large amount of government funds for the prevention and control of endemic arsenicosis.

Further Reading

1. Dongguang Wen, Fucun Zhang, Eryong Zhang, Cheng Wang, Shuangbao Han, Yan Zheng. Arsenic, fluoride and iodine in groundwater of China, Journal of Geochemical Exploration, 2013, 135, 1-21.

2. Rodríguez-Lado L, Sun G, Berg M, Zhang Q, Xue H, Zheng Q, Johnson CA. Groundwater arsenic contamination throughout china. Science, 2013, 341: 866-868.

3. Yu, G.Q., Sun, D.J., Zheng, Y., Health effects of exposure to natural arsenic in groundwater and coal in China: an overview of occurrence. Environ. Health Perspect, 2007, 115, 636-642.

4. Guifan Sun. Endemic arsenicosis: A clinical diagnostic manual with photo illustrations. Bangkok: UNCIF East Asia and Pacific Regional Office, 2004.

5. An D, Li D. Control status and countermeasures of endemic arsenicosis in Guizhou Province. Chin J Endemiol, 2005, 24(2): 214-216.

6. Liu J, Zheng B, Aposhian HV, Zhou Y, Chen ML, Zhang A, Waalkes MP. Chronic arsenic poisoning from burning high-arsenic-containing coal in Guizhou, China. Environ Health Perspect, 2002, 110(2): 119-122.

7. Rodríguez-Lado L, Sun G, Berg M, Zhang Q, Xue H, Zheng Q, Johnson CA. Groundwater arsenic contamination throughout china. Science, 2013, 341, 866-868.

8. Yang Kedi. Environmental Health. 7th edition. Beijing: People's Health Publishing House, 2012.

9. Sun D, Yu G, and Sun G. Pictorial manual for endemic arsenicosis diagnosis. Beijing: People's Medical Publishing House, 2015.

10. Yu GQ, Jun SD, Zheng Y. Health Effects of Exposure to Natural Arsenic in Groundwater and

Coal in China: An Overview of Occurrence, Environmental Health Perspectives, 2007, 115(4):
636-642

11. G. Sun. Arsenic contamination and arsenicosis in China. Toxicology and Applied Pharmacology,
2004, 198 (2) 268-271.

12. YL Jin, CK Liang, GL He, JX Cao, et al. Study on distribution of endemic arsenism in Chin.
Journal of Hygiene Research, 2003, 32(6): 519-540.

13. GQ Yu, Z Chen, LJ Zhao, DJ Sun. An analysis of the epidemic tendency of endemic arsenicosis
in China. Chin J Endemiol, 2010, 29(1): 3-8.

Chapter 5

Kashin-Beck Disease (KBD)

Xiong Guo, Feng Zhang, Xi Wang, Cuiyan Wu, Yujie Ning, Fangfang Yu, Mohammad Imran Younus, Mikko Juhani Lammi, Jun Yu, Hui Liu, Yanhong Cao

Abstract

Kashin-Beck disease (KBD) is an endemic chronic osteochondral disease, which has a high prevalence and morbidity in the Eastern Siberia of Russia, and in the broad diagonal, northern-east to southern-west belt in China and North Korea. In 1990's, it was estimated that in China 1.3 million patients had certain degree of symptoms of the disease, although even higher estimates have been presented. In China, the extensive prevalence peaked in the late 1950's, but since then, in contrast to the global trend of the osteoarthritis (OA), the number of cases has been dramatically falling. Up to 2013, there are 0.64 million patients with the KBD and 1.16 million at risk in 377 counties of 13 provinces or autonomous regions. This is obviously thanks to the preventive efforts carried out, including providing millions of people with dietary supplements and clean water, as well as relocating whole villages in China. However, relatively little is known about the environmental risk factors, and the rationale of the preventive effects and new data on a cellular and molecular level has begun to accumulate, which hopefully will uncover the grounds of the disease.

5.1 The Discovery of The Disease

In the nineteenth century, it was noticed that there were many patients, whose bones and joints were affected by serious joint pain, joint enlargements and deformations in the hand and limbs, and even more serious symptoms of dwarf deformities were observed in the patients of the northeastern to southwestern regions of China, in the southeastern Siberia in Russia, and in North Korea. However, the knowledge of the disease dated back to at least the sixteenth century. Globally, this kind of patients were mainly met in the two geographical belt regions, of which one was in the Eastern Asia district on the west coast of the Pacific Ocean (referred to as the "East Asian disease belt"), and the second in the north of Europe, from the Atlantic Ocean to the East Coast (referred to as "the Nordic disease belt"). According to reports, patients very similar to those described above appeared in the mountains in southwestern European countries, such as Portugal, France, Spain, Italy, and also Switzerland, in the western part of Russia and other Eastern European countries, but also in India and Africa, and North America bordering Canada. At that time, both residents and doctors did not know what kind of disease it was, or how to treat and prevent it. Generally, there were three sources of knowledge on how the disease was discovered: 1) not only from ancient medical books, but also from 2) the environmental, geographic and economic situation in the local county annals and 3) the legends among the local people in China, Russian and Japan. So, it is interesting to speculate when and where the disease came from.

5.1.1　The First Traces of Kashin-Beck Disease in China

KBD is a chronic endemic osteoarthropathy with a local distribution. Most patients suffer from morning stiffness of the joints, an arthritic pain without redness or heat, a limited motion and deformities of the affected joints, and in the most serious cases a retarded growth.

　　The KBD patients mainly have heavy cumbersome limbs, diffuse swelling joints for a long time, fixed joint pain with pain relief in daytime, while becoming more serious during the night, and pain relieved by warmth. Therefore, the traditional Chinese medicine calls the disease "the arthromyodynia" or "the bone-Bi-disease", which refers to the human body in an environment of cold wind at humid atmosphere, where the joint pain, invasion, numbness, flexion and extension conditions in limbs appear. It is interesting that the terms "the arthromyodynia" or "the bone-Bi-disease" are mentioned already in the "the Yellow Emperors Internal Classic", written in the period of Spring and Autumn and Warring States before BC 221. A similar description of this kind of disease, described as "Pain in many joints, body deformation and enlargement, and short and weak limbs", can be found in the Chinese medicine books titled "Jinkui yaolue" and "Treatise on cold pathogenic and miscellaneous diseases", written by a famous Chinese medical physician ZhongJing Zhang, who lived during the Han Dynasty 150-215 before AC.

In the year 1664 during the Ming Dynasty, a likely description of KBD appeared in the county record of Anze, Shanxi Province in the northern China, which is one of the areas of high prevalence of KBD. In 1908 during the Qing Dynasty, Liu Jianfeng (1865-1952), a member of demarcation Committee for Jilin and Shenyang, described the disease probably for the first time to exist in Chang Bai Mountain Jiang Gang of Jilin province, an endemic area located in the northeast of China. He described that many children, both boys and girls younger than 15-16 years old who lived in the mountain areas, appeared to have enlarged and shortened hands and feet, a limited motion of finger joints, and similar abnormalities also in the lower limbs. A detailed description of KBD was firstly reported by physician Fengshu Zhang in Jinlin Province in the northeast of China in 1934. He called the disease "Da Gujie Bing", which means "Big Bone disease", and suggested that it was the same disease as "Urov disease" in Russia. In 1956, Dr. N.I. ZhuravLev, medical scientists from the Soviet Union, confirmed that "Liu Guaizi Bing" in the Cuimu town of Linyou county in Shaanxi province was indeed the same disease.

Since the 1950's, the disease was investigated by Chinese scientists focusing on the epidemiology, clinical examination, radiology, pathology, biochemistry, molecular biology and medical geography as a common disease distributed from the north-east to the south-west of China, and they made their best efforts to study the etiology and pathogenesis of the disease, and how to control it.

5.1.2 The Discovery of Kashin-Beck Disease in Russia and Japan

In 1830, Irkustskian physician S.G. Filatov was the first to describe in a letter on the inhabitants in the eastern Zabaikaye, who were affected with pain and deformations in several joints. At that time, the name of the disease, which these inhabitants suffered from, was still undefined. Around the year 1836, M.A. Dokhturov, a physician from Nerchinsk, examined several patients who suffered from this disease and came from the areas along the bank of Urov river in the mountainous Transbaikal district, east of Lake Baikal in the Russian Siberia. The Urov river basin is one of the left-side tributaries of the Argun River, southeast of the Transbaikalia. The Argun river runs along the Chinese and Russian border in the north China's Inner Mongolia's Autonomous Region, and nurtures numerous wetlands in the region.

In 1849, a brief unsigned communication cited observation by a corresponding member Ivan. M. Yurensky, a land surveyor in Russian, who worked in this area and saw many patients who had similar changes of the hands and the limbs. He wrote a report to describe the main clinical manifestations of the disease, and showed the abnormal changes of the limbs' joints in some residents on the shore of the Urov river settlements. Some of them also suffered from the abnormally enlarged neck, and some hard-swollen mass growth out in the other part of the body. He stated that these patients had shortened fingers, a characteristic gait, and they could not either walk or work and live a normal life. Since I. M. Yurensky was a land surveyor in Nerchinsk, not a physician, he did not understand the nature of the disease. The affected people were mostly in their 20s, and sometimes younger, and had appearances of shortened fingers, bowing upper and lower limbs. When an unaffected girl or boy from the Urov river moved into another village along the river, they did not suffer from this disease, but the healthy children could develop joint deformities several years after migration to the diseased areas. The pastureland in these areas was poor, and the marshes were covered with rust. Sheep and a few horses were the mainly domestic animals.

In 1856, seven years after the Yurensky's reporter, Zabaikalye Cossack military detachment was established in this area. The military headquarters soon found out that it was difficult to recruit the soldiers from some segments in this region due to the body deformities in the local population. Cossacks, kazaki were a group of predominantly East Slavic people who became known as members of democratic, semi-military communities, predominantly located in Ukraine and in Russia. They inhabited sparsely populated areas and islands in the lower Dnieper, Don, Terek, and Urov river basins, and played an important role in the historical and cultural development of both Russia and Ukraine.

Due to the difficulties in the recruitment of the soldiers in the Urov river shore, a special order from the headquarters of Zabaikalye Cossack military was issued to investigate this problem to understand what reasons caused the disease of the body deformity in the local population. The investigating duties were assigned to Nicholas I. Kashin (N. I. Kashin, 1825-1872), a military doctor of the 4th infantry battalion in Cossack brigade at Olochinsk on the Argun river. He was born in the central Russia in 1825 and worked mostly in the eastern Siberia. He studied medicine in Moscow from 1846 to 1851. He then served in the army for ten years to repay the costs of his education, since his father, a feldsher, was unable to afford the tuition for him. Kashin was the author of some 60 publications, two of which dealt with osteoarthropathy. Following the service in Siberia, Kashin worked at the Military Academy in Moscow in 1861 and wrote a doctoral thesis on a subject unrelated to Urov disease. In 1864, he returned to Irkutsk as a civilian medical inspector.

On April 24, 1856, he was directed to investigate the health problem at the Urov river shore and examine the patients, their hygienic condition and occupational environment, and the living conditions of the local people. At the beginning, he considered these abnormalities might be an adult form of the English disease rickets. A month later, Kashin drafted a report to the chief ataman of the Cossacks entitled "Description of endemic goiter and other diseases prevailing along the Urov River". Kashin draw up a picture of a Cossack who had both a large goiter and deformed extremities, leaning on a walking stick. He interpreted that these skeletal abnormalities could be one manifestation of complex systemic disturbances following prolonged fever, scurvy, syphilis, and hereditary predispositions. Since the disease had an endemic distribution, spreading in the areas of The Urov and Uryumkan rivers, the disease was named the Urov disease.

In 1899 - 1902, Eugene V Beck (1885-1916), a junior physician in Chita and the district officer of the Fourth Medical Department of the Transbaikal Cossack Army, found similar patients in other settlements located in the tributaries of the Shilka and Argun rivers, including the Gazimur, the Unda and the upper and middle Borzya. He organized an epidemic investigation in 11 villages close to Nerchinsk city, assisted by his wife, A. N. Beck. After examination of 1009 patients out of 3153 inhabitants, including children in the families of the patients with deformed, enlarged joints and limping gait, Beck gave this disease a name "osteoarthritis deformans endemic". This term is very similar to the endemic bone and joint disease used at present, and describes the clinical manifestations at the advanced stage of this disease. Beck stated in 1903 that the prevalence ranged from 6.5% to 46.5%, with an average rate of 31.6% in these endemic areas, and the regions were classified as the high prevalence type areas of this disease.

Following his investigation and the permission from the Chief Military Inspector, Beck transferred six Cossack subjects aged from 16 to 23 to the Clinical Military Hospital in St. Petersburg for the systematic anthropological, radiological, and neuropsychiatric examinations in October 1903. In 1906, Beck wrote his doctoral thesis based on the above investigation in St. Petersburg Academy, and published it in a German journal Archive für Klinische Chirurgie in 1908. Beck considered then that the skeletal deformities of the disease were specific changes, rather than a manifestation of a multifactorial systemic disorder, which was Kashin's understanding. Based on his investigation, Beck thought that the disease may be related to poor drinking water, but did not understand what the noxious agent could be. After the sudden death of Dr. Beck, his wife A. N. Beck continued to study the anthropometric changes of the disease, and published the results in 1927. Based on the Beck's idea, she wanted to solve which opinion, i.e., the idea of a systemic disease by Kashin or the specific skeletal disorder by Beck, was reasonable for the disease. She also designed the experimental prevention to observe the effect of boiling the drinking water to kill and eliminate its possible infective agents. Following the above investigations by Drs. Kashin and Beck with his wife, the Urov disease was studied by many local physicians and professors.

The third pathway to discovery of the Kashin-Beck disease came from the medical scientists from Japan. In 1919, Dr. Ikano, an army surgeon, noted that some patients in the northern part of the Korean Peninsula suffered from a chronic bone and joints disease with deformed limbs, and considered their clinical manifestations similar to Kashin-Beck disease. In 1927, Dr. Nakamura examined these kinds of patients also in the southern part the Korean Peninsula. During the years 1928 to 1929, Drs. Kato and Kim observed some patients who suffered from abnormal manifestations similar to Kashin-Beck disease in the above-mentioned areas. In the early 1930s, professor Tokio Takamori and his colleagues from the former Manchuria Medical College described the disease distribution, clinical features, radiology and pathological anatomy at the General Congress of the Japanese Society of Internal Endemic Occurrence of KBD in the northeastern China. From these description, Kashin-Beck disease was shown to be distributed in the northern part of the Korean Peninsula and the northeastern China, which were close to the endemic areas of the southern Siberia in 1940's, as shown in the book "Kashin-Beck's disease" written by Dr Tokio Takamori in 1968.

5. 1. 3 The Reason Why We Call It "Kashin-Beck Disease"

The disease has been known worldwide as Kashin-Beck disease in honors of the contribution of Drs. Kashin and Beck with his wife for their description and study on the characteristics of the clinical manifestations and the epidemic situation in the early disease history, even though many non-scientific and scientific names have been suggested since the disease discovery. In 1928, Kashin-Beck disease already appeared in a title of the etiology of Kashin-Beck disease (osteochondrous deformans) in Zabajkal by V. G Sipacev. However, Kashin-Beck disease is often misspelled "Kaschin-Beck disease" in English publications and books. This confusion was clearly described by Prof Sokoloff in 1989 pointing out that is an inappropriate carryover from the German transliteration of the Cyrillic, comparing to "Kashin-Becksche Krankheit" in German.

In the beginning, the non-scientific name was popular in the publications and books over the scientific name, but it is used as the specific scientific name now. Before the name of Kashin-Beck disease, the first non-scientific name was "Urov disease" in Russia, since this disease was discovered in the Urov river basin. Later, it was called "Kashin's disease" and "Beck's disease" after Drs Kashin and Beck who studied the disease. In China, the disease was called "Da Gu-Jie Bing" or "big bone joint disease" and "liǔ guǎi zi bìng". The latter refers to the deformed joints of this disease, which reminds a bending with deformed willow, pronounced as "liǔ guǎi zi bìng" in Chinese.

Table 5.1 shows the development of the scientific name of Kashin-Beck disease from the early stage from 1859 to until now. It was considered as a chronic, endemic, degeneration and deformed osteoarthritis from Eugene V. Beck from 1906 to 1936, and showed mainly the changes in the advanced stage of the disease. Also in 1936, professor Kubo in Japan considered the disease as dystrophic, but not infective, disease, and he suggested that the disease was endemic deformed osteoarthritis resulted in the name osteoarthropathia deformans endemic. In 1943, Sergiycvski and Rubinstein in Russia proposed this disease was a food fusariotoxicosis, which selectively impairs the endochondral ossification in the skeletal system. In 1968, Takamori Tokio in his book "Kashin-Beck's disease" proposed the disease was enchondral dysostosis, which affects metaphyseal longitudinal and epiphyseal transverse growth and is characterized by endemic occurrence without genetic factors. In 1975, World Health Organization classified this disease as the other specific arthropathies in International Classification of Diseases, Revision 10 in 1989. In 1990, the name acquired chondronecrosis was proposed by Leon Sokoloff in USA in 1990, and osteochondrosis endemica humanis by Dongxu Mo in PR of China in 1994, due to comparable pathological changes with animal osteochondrosis. The name KBD was classified as endemic deformed osteoarthrosis by Ministry of Health, PR China in 1993, and osteoarthritis deformans endemica by international classification for bone diseases in 2004.

Table 5.1　The list of the disease name for Kashin-Beck Disease with its reporters

The diseases names were suggested for Kashin-Beck disease	reporters	year
A complication of endemic goiter	Kashin N.I.	1859
Osteoarthritis deforman endemic	Beck E.B.	1906
Chronic progressive polyosteoathrititis	Okano. T.A	1919
Endemic osteochondritis	Dobrovolsky LO	1925
Osteoarthropathia deformans endemic	Kubo H	1936
Panarthritis deformans endemic	Hiyeda K	1936
Food fusariotoxicosis	Sergiycvski, Rubinstein	1943
Dysostosis enchondrosis endemic/Dysostosis encho-ndrosis meta-epiphysis	Takamori Tokio	1943

Continue

The diseases names were suggested for Kashin-Beck disease	reporters	year
Degenerative arthropathy	Sella EJ	1973
Osteodysplasia congenital	Poznanski AK	1974
Other specific arthropathies (Kashin-Beck Disease)	WHO, World Health Organization	1975
Endemic chromic osteoarthrosis	Peipu Yin	1983
Endemic osteoarthrophy with unknown cause	Nutrition, USA	1987
Spondyloepiphyseal dysostosis,	Beighton P	1988
Epidemic osteoarthrosis	Rheumatological Association, Russian	1988
M12 Other specific arthropathies (Kashin-Beck Disease)	International Classifi-cation of Diseases,Revision 10	1989
Acquired chondronecrosis	Sokoloff L	1990
Exopathic bone metabolism impair or dystrophy	Zhizhong Qian	1991
Osteochondrosis endemica humanis	Dongxu Mo	1994
Endemic deformed osteoarthrosis	Ministry of Health, PR China	1994
Osteoarthritis deformans endemica	Classification for bone disease	2004

5.2 Epidemiology and Disease Characteristics

5.2.1 Which Regions Are Involved in The Occurrence of KBD

In recent decades, Kashin-Beck disease is mainly distributed in China within a narrow zone from the northeast to the southwest, involving Beijing, Heilongjiang, Jilin, Liaoning, Hebei, Shandong, Henan, Inner Mongolia, Shanxi, Shaanxi, Gansu, Sichuan, Qinghai, Tibet and certain other places. The northeast parts extend to minority areas of Siberia and the northern parts in North Korea.

5.2.2 What Kind of People is More Susceptible to KBD

Kashin-Beck disease occurs mainly in children and adolescents, and there are a few new cases in adults. In high prevalence areas, children at the age of 2-3 years old may be suffered to the disease, while in mild prevalence areas, the age of the onset can be delayed until the age over ten.

5. 2. 3 What is the Climate and Geography of KBD Areas

In the northwest Loess Plateau KBD endemic areas of China, the incidence of KBD in gully regions is higher than that in the northeast of China. The terrain of KBD endemic areas are mostly shallow mountains areas and hills, in which the onset of KBD is the most serious in low-lying moist areas, such as river valleys and intermountain valleys. However, the relationship between the incidence and the terrain is relatively variable, since some villages with high number of KBD cases also can be found in several plain areas, such as Songnen Plain and Songliao Plain. All the KBD endemic areas are located in the border regions of the south-eastern coastal hot-moist monsoon regions and the northwest drought-cold inland, where are belong to continental climate zone with short summer season, long frost season, and an obvious temperature difference between day and night.

5. 2. 4 What is the Problem Faced by KBD Patients in Their Daily Life

Clinically, KBD patients can be classified into three levels from Degree I to Degree III. The patients at Degree I usually had multiple symmetric thickening finger joints and thickening limb joints with a limited range of motion, pain, and light muscle atrophy. Degree II classicfication is based on Degree I, but the symptoms and signs are worse. There is an appearance of short (toe) deformities, short limb deformities and short stature. In degree III, the symptoms and signs are even worse, including short limb deformities and short stature. When the disease is in degree I, it can be stopped if separated from the ward. In degree II, the prognosis is better if the epiphyseal plates do not continue calcifying or ossifying and not expanding the scope. In degree III, the epiphyseal plate has been ossified, which is difficult to recover. Kashin Beck disease has no direct threat to life, and it does not directly affect the lifetime, but the impact on the labor force is huge, the severe cases not only lose the ability to work, but also the ability to take care of themselves.

5.2.5   Is the Number of KBD Patients in China Increasing or Decreasing

According to the stastistics of the 2014 "national survey focused on prevention and control of endemic diseases", there are a total of 6111887 patients with KBD. Due to a decreasing annual incidence of new patients and deaths of the older patients, the number of KBD patients had a decreasing trend. According to the surveillance data. The detection rate of new KBD cases was decreased year by year. The X ray average detection rate was 0.17% in 2015 (Fig.5.1). Results of "the National Endemic Disease Control, the 12th Five-Year Plan" show that more than 95% of the investigated endemic KBD villages of China have achieved the control level.

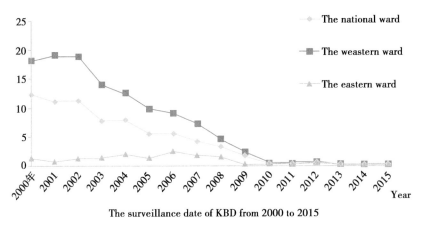

The surveillance date of KBD from 2000 to 2015

Fig. 5.1   The surveillance date of KBD from 2000 to 2015

5.3   Etiology and Epidemic Mechanism

5.3.1   The Etiology of KBD

Several hypotheses have been proposed on the etiology of KBD in the past 150 years, including calcium deficiency, sulphur deficiency, and excess of strontium in combination with deficiency of calcium, fungal (fusarium oxysporum) toxin in cereal, and high humic acids in drinking water. Up to now, three major environmental hypotheses have been under debate for KBD: (1) serious cereal contamination, such as T-2 toxin, by mycotoxin-producing fungi, (2) selenium deficiency, (3) hypothesis of high humic acid levels in the drinking water. Recently, the multifactorial model with interactions of environment and its responsive genes has been considered for KBD.

5.3.2 What is the Relationship between Grain Mildew and Fungi in Occurrence with KBD

Hypothesis of cereal contamination by mycotoxin-producing fungi was originally put forward by the former Soviet Union in 1943-1945. This theory showed that certain fusarium contaminated the grains harvested in KBD area and produced heat-resistant mycotoxins, as well as other second metabolites in the grains. Residents who consumed this kind of food chronically would suffer KBD. During 1932-1945, the Soviet Union scholars F. P. Sergievsky, Y. I. Rubinstein and others found that grains grown in KBD area were the main source of the pathogenic factor. In the process of harvest, threshing, drying and storage, the grains were contaminated by fungi, and mycotoxins were produced under the humid conditions. In some KBD areas, oxysporum as the preponderant fusarium tainted the wheat field and produced the mycotoxins, which selectively damaged the osteoepiphysis and advance the development of deformed endochondral bone. So, KBD is also called "Food Mycotoxic Enchondral Osteodystrophy".

The main evidences supporting the hypothesis are: (1) based on the distribution of KBD in the former Soviet Union and China, all the KBD areas belong to the continental climate (short summer, long frost period, obvious temperature difference between day and night). Harvest of the grains occurs in the rainy season, which is suitable for fungi proliferation, (2) many dominant fungi are detected from the food produced in the KBD areas. For example, in Chita of the former Soviet Union, the preponderant fungus is Fusarium Sporotrichiella. Var. Poae. In the northeast of China, Fusarium oxysporum is dominant; in Shaanxi, Fusarium Graminearum and Fusarium moniliforme; and in Gansu, Alternaria alternata. (3) Compared with the non-KBD areas, the KBD areas have higher concentration of mycotoxins, which are Butenolide, Alternariol methyl ether, Deoxynivalenol, 15-Deoxy-nivalenol, 3-Deoxynivalenol, and Nivalenol, respectively. (4) The study of chondrocytes cultured in vitro proved that mycotoxins, such as Butenolide, Deoxynivalenol, Nivalenol, not only induce chondrocytes' dedifferentiation and apoptosis, but also inhibit their DNA synthesis and cell proliferation. They also result in the damage of chondrocyte membrane system, including cell membrane, nuclear membrane and all organelles, triggering the metabolic disorder biochemically. Using extracts from Fusarium sporotrichioides or Fusarium oxysporum to feed rats and dogs, cartilage lesions in these experimental animals were similar to those seen in KBD. (5) In Shuangyashan City, Heilongjiang province (1972-1980) and Fusong County, Jilin province (1958-1965), trials of changing staple food for prevention and control of KBD obtained effective preventive effect. In Shangzhi County, Heilongjiang province (1970-1988), a field test of planting rice and consuming rice as staple food for control of KBD also obtained effective preventive effect.

In 1990s, Professor Jianbo Yang proposed that T-2 toxin was the pathogenic factor of KBD (Fig.5.2). The main evidences are as below: (1) It is not until the middle of 1990s that the phenomenon of T-2 toxin accumulating extraordinarily in grains and corn produced in KBD's areas was revealed. T-2 toxin was detected from the wheat flour consumed by the KBD families using ELISA technique, and the content of T-2 toxin was obviously higher than that in the wheat flour consumed by the non-KBD families. Levels of T-2 toxin in the grains harvested in KBD area should be below 100 µg/kg, or at least below 300 µg/kg, to prevent KBD.

(2) Feeding chickens with food, to which T-2 toxin was added to reach 100 µg/kg per day for 3-5 weeks, caused chickens' pathological changes that were similar to KBD. Feeding chickens with food, in which fusarium-contaminated ground grain was added at a ratio of one tenth, also had the similar result. (3) T-2 toxin had obvious inhibitory effect on the proliferation and DNA synthesis of chondrocytes, and the effect was positively associated with the concentration of T-2 toxin. The T-2 toxin could induce apoptosis and dedifferentiation in chondrocytes cultured

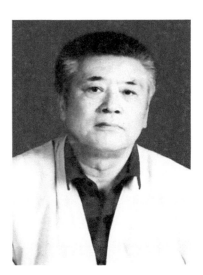

Fig. 5.2   Professor Jianbo Yang

in vitro. The route of transmission and carriers of KBD causative agent is illustrated in Fig.5.3.

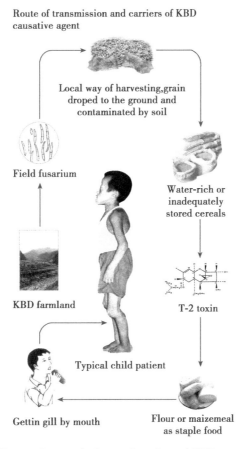

Route of transmission and carriers of KBD causative agent

Local way of harvesting,grain droped to the ground and contaminated by soil

Field fusarium

Water-rich or inadequately stored cereals

KBD farmland

T-2 toxin

Typical child patient

Gettin gill by mouth

Flour or maizemeal as staple food

Fig. 5.3　Route of transmission and carriers of KBD causative agent

5.3.3　Which Element's Deficiency Causes KBD

More than 50 suspicious pathogenic factors causing KBD have been proposed by scientists in the past 150 years. One of them is the biogeochemical hypothesis, which suggest that the occurrence and development of KBD are related to the specific ecological geographical conditions. Overload, lack or disproportionality of some chemical elements in the KBD endemic environment have been considered to influence the normal metabolism of minerals in vivo, possibly leading to KBD. Based on the imbalance of various trace elements in soil, water and crop in KBD endemic areas, a former Soviet Union scientist A. P. Vinogradov first proposed the biogeochemical hypothesis during 1939 to 1949. In the following research from 1949 to 1973, professor V. V. Kovalsky considered that the low contents of strontium, barium, calcium, phosphorus, potassium and sodium in the water, soil and residents' dietary might result in KBD.

In 1970s, Chinese scientist found that the environmental selenium (Se) deficiency was closely associated with KBD, and gradually developed the selenium deficiency hypothesis for KBD. The main evidence of selenium deficiency hypothesis for KBD is as follows: firstly, the low level of selenium in the external environment of KBD endemic area lead to the Se-low nutrition state of the human body in residents via the food chain in KBD endemic areas. The distribution of KBD endemic areas almost shares the same zone with the distribution of Se-low soil. The total content of Se in most soil of endemic area was less than 0.15 mg/kg, less than 0.02 mg/kg in the grain, and contents of Se in the soil, wheat and corn in KBD endemic areas were significantly less than those of the non-KBD endemic areas. Second, the Se contents of blood, urine and hair of children in KBD endemic areas were lower than those in non-KBD endemic areas. Based on the selenium deficiency in vivo in the patients, they had series of metabolic changes, such as decreased activity of GSH-PX in the whole blood, the increased activity of GOT, GPT, LDH, HBDH, LPO, and free fat content in serum. Thirdly, the epidemiological investigation suggested that there was a negative correlation between Se level and prevalence of KBD. Finally, the prevalence of children KBD can be diminished after selenium supplement. For example, new prevalence of KBD was 0.45% after selenium supplement in 9343 normal children cases in KBD endemic areas, while prevalence of KBD was 1.95% in the 2963 normal children cases with non-selenium supplement in endemic areas at same period. During the period of 1975 to 1979, Se contents in hair and urine of 400 KBD children (hair: 59 ± 25 ng/g to 98±24 ng/g; urine: 2.09±0.81 μg/24 h to 2.88 ± 1.20 μg/24 h) in Shaanxi province in northwestern China were much lower than those of the healthy children in non-KBD areas (hair: 195±54 ng/g to 343±124 ng/g; urine: 5.08±1.13 μg/24 h to 7.22 ± 1.93 μg/24 h). The Se deficiency had continued for decades in Shaanxi, Sichuan, Tibet, and other endemic provinces of China. The low internal Se level (e.g., in hair and urine) was consistent with the low Se content in the soil (1.04-4.30 ng/g), wheat (27-31 ng/g), corn (20-23 ng/g) and drinking water (0.12-0.32 ng/g).

Besides the Se deficiency, iodine (I) levels are also low in the KBD endemic areas. Epidemiological investigation suggested that most Se deficiency areas overlap with I deficiency areas. The distribution of KBD endemic areas was consistent with serious endemic areas of iodine deficiency disease, and the distribution of cretinism, caused by serious lack of I, was highly consistent with KBD endemic areas. Survey results of Se and I level of children in Tibetian KBD endemic areas suggested that 49% of the children suffered from KBD, 46% from goiter, and 1% from cretinism. Urine iodine levels of 66% of the children in endemic areas were less than 2 μg/dl, and urine iodine contents of the patients with KBD were significantly lower than those in control group. Therefore, I is still a risk factor of KBD in the serious Se deficiency areas of KBD endemic areas.

5.3.4   Whether the KBD is Related to Drinking Water or Not

A high content of humic acids in the drinking water is another environmental risk factor candidate in the past 150 years since it was found, although the cause of KBD is still unclear. At the early stage, Chang Bai Mountain area is one of the KBD prevalence areas geographically located in the east of China. In 1908, Liu Jianfeng, a local administrator, made a statement on KBD in a book named "A Brief of River and Ridge in Chang Bai Mountain". He wrote, "The walnut trees behind the ridge are most harmful to human beings. Branches, leaves, flowers, fruits roots and barks decay in the mountain year after year out of rain and snow immersion. The produced poisonous gas is carried in water along the brooklets to the river and diffuses into wells and springs. People dwelling in the mountain suffered from shortening of hands and feet, enlargement of joints of fingers and toes from the age below 15-16 years of both males and females. It is still harmful to the people. Half of the victims drink mountain water and half drink river water. Few of them have wells and occasionally a shallow well less than 5 feet deep can be found. It is not surprising that there are so many victims." Finally, he pointed out, "Only by drilling deep well, can people be protected" (Liu, 1908). The following is a summary of our studies on the relationship between KBD and drinking water in supporting the above statement.

The geographical distribution of KBD covered an oblique belt running from northeast to southwest area in China, especially in western provinces, such as Shannxi Provence, Sichuan Provence, Qinghai Provence and Tibet Provence. The western regions are relatively arid regions in China, for example, the water consumption per capita of residents in Shaanxi Province is only one quarter of the national average value, and in some towns, the value is even less than one-sixth. However, the local precipitation is not such little in rainy season. Thus, to solve drinking water problem, the villagers will collect and store rainwater in pits during the rainy season, whereby water that local residents eat is also known as "pit-water"

The pit is a common water storage structure in arid and semi-arid regions. It is dug into the shape of well under the thick layer of a mountain plateau area. It is built with anti-seepage facilities to store runoff water, such as rain, snow or other precipitations, among which rain is the main source. Yet, rain is easily polluted in the process of precipitation by all kinds of substances in the atmosphere, thus, common pollutants in the atmosphere are likely to be contained in the rain. The pollutants include sulphurous acid or sulfuricacid transformed from sulfurdioxide or sulfurtrioxide in the air and dissolved in water, soil derived mineral ions like Al^{3+}, Ca^{2+}, Mg^{2+}, Fe^{3+}, gas transformations like SO_4^{2-}, NO^-, NH^{4+}, H^+, anthropogenic emissions like Cr, Zn, Cu, Pb, organic-like organic acids alkanes, aromatic hydrocarbons, photochemical reaction product like PAN, and non-dissolved substance from fuel combustion.

Pit-water is usually in a static state, basically with little or no flow, thus, the water does not have self-purification ability. Long period of static state forms a special environment inside the water, causing a large number of microbes to reproduce, the lack of dissolved oxygen, the exceeding of sensory index and other water deterioration phenomenon. Substances like dry branches and fallen leaves, human and animal excreta, or household garbage, if they exist in the process of gathering water, will make the total number of biological oxygen demand, and the number of coliform bacteria in the water cellar to exceed safety value. Shaanxi Provinceis in Loess Plateau area. Due to poor structure of loess, special geological and geomorphological conditions with weak anti-dispersion ability, as well as low vegetation coverage rate, concentrated rainfall, soil and water loss, water turbidity and suspended particles in the water of the Loess Plateau area have increased after part of the sediment flows into water.

Later, studies have reported that the incidence of KBD is related to the drinking water. Humic acid content in drinking water in KBD area is significantly higher than that in non-endemic areas. The content of some trace elements in the drinking water, such as selenium and zinc, is lower than those in non-endemic areas. The villagers' drinking water in Rangtang County of Aba prefecture of Sichuan Province, a rare KBD endemic area in China, is mainly from the gully surface water, shallow groundwater of Du river and Zequ river. The major source of the water is from precipitation and snowmelt. According to the investigation and analysis of main drinking water quality, its mineralization and hardness degree are quite low, while the content of humic acid is more than 2 mg/l, and the indicator of coliform bacteria is much higher than national standard. (The indicator is back to normal after the water is boiled.) Among these factors, high level of humic acid is considered to be one of the causes for chondrocytes degeneration and cartilage damage. Humic acid is the organic substance produced and accumulated by decomposition and transformation of microorganisms of the remains of animals and plants, especially the plants. In northeastern China, plateau is the main topography. It has bountiful forest and grassland, lofty mountains, and high vegetation cover rate, thus, humic acid is easily formed and accumulated.

After knowing the relationship between KBD and drinking water, local residents and the government began to pay attention to water sanitation and water quality improvement. On one hand, the plants, garbage etc. were prevented from entering the pit in the process of pit-water collection. On the other hand, the residents made their best not to drink pit-water. Because there is a strange phenomenon "healthy island" in KBD area ("healthy island" is one place within KBD prevalence area, but without KBD patients), the residents in prevalence area took water from the healthy island nearby. The government has also invested a lot of manpower, finance and material resources to drinking water improvement projects in KBD area, for example, groundwater exploitation and division, groundwater supply project, dynamic surveillance system of water quantity, and water quality and migration project. Based on the government projects, the residents in KBD area can use running water. Migration project has moved residents scatteredly living in highland, caves, mountain and other similar places to new villages built by government with great living facilities. Aba Tibetan and Qiang Autonomous Prefecture is in the northwest of Sichuan Province, with most ethnic minority population. Aba has 1352 villages, in which there are 379 villages having KBD patients. The number of patients has reached 40,000 people, up to a quarter of the total population. Through the migration project, most pastoralists have lived in new, spacious and clean houses until recent years (Fig. 5. 4).

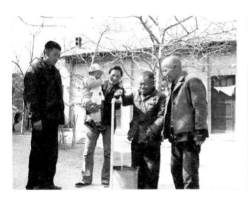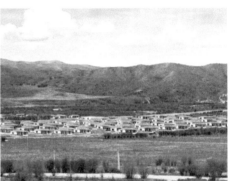

Fig. 5.4　The villagers happily look the clean tap water flowing out (left). The new village for herdsmen in Hongyuan County, Aba Tibetan and Qiang Autonomous Prefecture benefit from government's migration project (right).

In conclusion, drinking water increases the risk of KBD in endemic areas. The water can be the medium of selenium deficiency, contaminated by fungal mycotoxins, and enriched with humic acids. Through the improved nutritional diets, the living environment and the quality of drinking water in the KBD areas, KBD has been effectively prevented.

5. 3. 5　Are There any Abnormal Genes and Proteins Involved in KBD

5. 3. 5. 1　Abnormally Expressed Genes in KBD Articular Cartilage

The gene expression patterns of articular cartilage and peripheral blood mononuclear cells of KBD patients are significantly different from that of healthy people. Using human whole genome expression chip, 55 up-regulated genes and 24 down-regulated genes were identified in KBD articular chondrocytes. 79 genes were expressed at abnormal levels to participate in various cell processes, mainly including metabolism, apoptosis, cell proliferation and matrix degradation. Additionally, gene expression of peripheral blood mononuclear cells showed 97 abnormal genes in KBD patients. The 83 genes were differently expressed. Their function involved apoptosis, metabolism, immunity, cytoskeleton, cell movement and extracellular matrix. The above gene expression analysis results suggest that chondrocyte metabolism and apoptosis related genes contribute to the articular cartilage damage of KBD (Fig. 5.5).

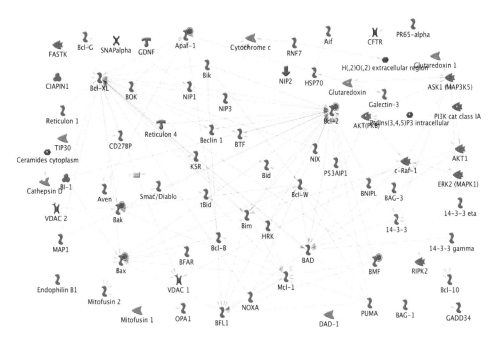

Fig. 5.5　Interaction network of Kashin-Beck disease chondocyte gene compared with the normal individual analyzed by Transcriptome Browser software. Twenty significant genes are involved in the network. Different cytoarchitectures are denoted by different colors.

To reveal the mechanism of differently expressed genes involved in the development of KBD, gene set-based pathway expression analysis approach was applied to the gene expression studies of KBD. Researchers found that apoptosis-related, hypoxia-related and mitochondria-related pathways were significantly abnormally expressed in KBD articular cartilage. For instance, pathway for apoptosis was found to be highly expressed in KBD articular cartilage. This pathway acts in response to various types of intracellular stress, including growth factor withdrawal, DNA damage, unfolding stresses in the endoplasmic reticulum and death receptor stimulation. Following the reception of stress signals, proapoptotic BCL-2 family proteins are activated, and subsequently inactivate antiapoptotic BCL-2 proteins. This interaction leads to the release of apoptotic factors, and ultimately results in cell death.

5.3.5.2 *Abnormally Expressed Proteins in KBD Articular Cartilage*

There are also significant differences in protein expression patterns between KBD patients and healthy people. Using protein mass spectra analytic technique, researchers identified 11 protein peaks differentially expressed between KBD and healthy subjects. For instance, the expression of a protein peak with m/z 15886 was significantly decreased in KBD patients compared to healthy subjects. In contrast, the expression of the protein peaks with m/z 2952 and 3400 were significantly increased in KBD patients compared to healthy subjects. The identified abnormal proteins can be used as disease biomarkers for diagnosing KBD. Using classification tree, researchers identified three potential protein biomarkers at 5336, 6880 and 4155 m/z. The sensitivity and specificity of the three protein biomarkers achieved 86.36 % and 88.89 % for distinguishing KBD from healthy subjects. To reveal the mechanism of differently expressed proteins involved in the cartilage damage of KBD, researchers further compared the protein expression patterns of KBD chondrocytes and healthy chondrocytes. They identified 38 abnormally expressed protein spots in KBD chondrocytes (Fig. 5.6). The identified differential expression proteins functionally involved in protein metabolism, chondrocyte structural abnormalities and oxidative stress. The above results support the presence of abnormal synthesis, metabolism, subcellular localization and molecular functions of proteins in KBD chondrocytes.

5.3.6 Is KBD Infective or Hereditary

5.3.6.1 *Virus Infection and KBD*

HPVB19 virus was first discovered in 1975 by Australian virologist Yvonne Cossart.

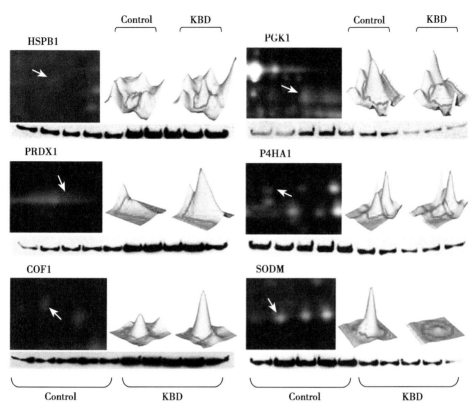

Fig. 5.6　(A) DIGE gel images of high abundance HSPB1, PRDX1, and COF1 labeled with Cy5 represent KBD; and high abundance PGK1, P4HA1, and SODM labeled with Cy3 represent the healthy control. (B) Three-dimensional visualization of HSPB1, PRDX1, COF1, PGK1, P4HA1, and SODM abundance in KBD and healthy control samples. (C) Western blot analysis of HSPB1, PRDX1, COF1, PGK1, P4HA1, and SODM levels in KBD and healthy control samples from group 2.

In 1985, White and Reid found that HPVB19 infection could result in arthritis resembling symptoms, including joint pain, stiff and swelling. Women are approximately twice as likely as men to experience arthritis after HPVB19 infection. Typically, joint symptoms disappear after 1-3 weeks, but in some cases, they may last weeks to months. Bi et al. reported that he observed inclusion bodies in the necrotic chondrocytes of KBD patients. Inclusion body is nuclear or cytoplasmic aggregate of stainable substances, which often indicates viral multiplication in a bacterium or a eukaryotic cell. Bi et al. inferred that KBD was caused by virus infection. Another study also reported that children＇s infection rates of HPVB19 virus in KBD prevalent areas were higher than those in non-KBD prevalent areas. However, the endemic characteristics of KBD does not support virus infection hypothesis. The experimental evidence linking KBD to HPVB19 virus infection is also limited. Currently, it is generally accepted that HPVB19 virus infection is not one of the major environmental causes of KBD.

5.3.6.2 *Genetic Susceptibility and KBD*

Although KBD is regarded as an environmental disease, there is an increased evidence supporting the impact of genetic factors on the risk of KBD. It has long been observed that not all families or family members suffered from KBD, even if they lived at the same environment in KBD prevalent areas. Under the same environmental condition, the individual difference in KBD susceptibility suggested roles of genetic factors in the development of KBD. It was also found that the parents and siblings of KBD index cases have a 3-4 times higher risk of KBD than random unrelated individuals. However, previous KBD researchers have not been able to clarify the genetic basis of KBD due to technical limitations.

With the rapid advances of genetics and molecular biology, a group of genetic studies have been conducted, confirming the significant impact of genetic susceptibility on the risk of KBD. Lu et. al analyzed 10,823 subjects from 1,361 families and observed significant familial aggregation of KBD patients. They suggested that more than 40% risk of KBD could be explained by genetic factors. Using linkage analysis approach, Ren et al. identified 6 KBD-related loci at chromosome 2, 6 and 12. Using a more accurate genetic association analysis approach, researchers identified multiple KBD-associated susceptibility genes, including HLA-DRB1, ABI3BP, GPX1, GPX4, ITPR2 and TNF genes (Fig. 5.7). However, the KBD risk explained by these identified susceptibility genes is limited, suggesting the existence of undiscovered susceptibility genes.

Although the importance of genetic factors in the development of KBD has been demonstrated, most researchers believe that KBD is an environmental disease. The genes can affect the progress of KBD through altering individual susceptibility to environmental risk factors. However, the mechanism of joint effects between environmental risk factors and susceptibility genes need more studies.

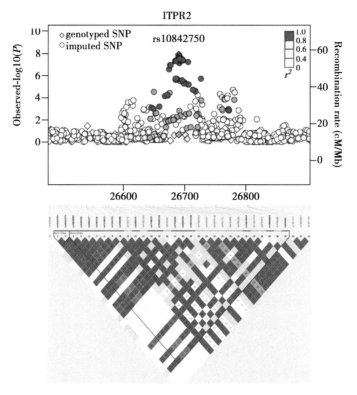

Fig. 5.7   Regional association plot (top) and linkage disequilibrium (LD) map (bottom) of ITPR2. The - log10 (P) value of each genotyped or imputed single-nucleotide polymorphism (SNP) is plotted against chromosomal positions in a 400-kb region centered on rs10842750. The right y-axis presents the estimated genetic recombination rate (1000 Genomes Project, Phase 1 integrated data, version 3). The LD map is based on HapMap genotype data for Han Chinese.

5.4   Clinical Manifestation and Diagnosis

5.4.1   What Are the Clinical Manifestations of KBD

Kashin-Beck disease progression is relatively slow, at the early stage of the onset, most patients did not have obvious symptoms, although thickening and deformation in finger joints, ankle, or elbow have often been in unconsciously present. Some patients will feel weak, are easy to get exhausted, suffer from inappetence and muscle aches. Their arms and legs may have a feeling that the ants crawling on, or numbness. In the endemic area where the pathogenic factors are active, most patients have painful joints of the limb as a main symptom. After getting up in the morning, adult KBD patients whose limb joint are stiff and painful, have difficulties to move. However, after light activities, the pain may be eased. Also, if a few "Tieguaizi" patients take part in physical labor, they may not feel the pain. The more critically ill the patients are, the more difficulties they have in walking and squatting, with staggering gait or walking which resembles duck walking. Individual case has the symptoms of joint interlocking, which may be caused by intra-articular loose body.

5.4.2 What Are the Signs of KBD

In the early stage patients' fingers can bend slightly to the palm side, the distal finger looking like a goose head droop. The result of disease progression is joint enlargement, deformation, dyskinesia and muscle atrophy. It begins in the fingers, toes and ankles, wrists, and metacarpophalangeal joints, followed by elbow and knee joints. In the most severe late stage, the patients shoulder, hip and spine joints may show hyperplasia deformations and dyskinesia. Heberden's nodes, which are bony swelling especially in the distal interphalangeal joint, often develop in KBD. The wrist can be flat and broad or narrow thick, tilt to the ulnar or lateral deflection, styloid process of ulna up-lift, which is so-called Medalens malformation. The thickening elbow joint is curve buckling, knee joints get thickened, and it is possible to see "X" or "O" shaped legs. The ankle is thick, just like toe joint. The thickened joint has activity limitation, and the motion range is smaller than that before sickness.

The greater thenar and hypothenar muscle, biceps, triceps, and gastrocnemius muscle atrophies are also observed. Severe patients have short fingers, short limb deformity, dislocated or subluxated fingers, toes, wrist, elbow, knee, and ankle joints. Often the height of patients is not commensurate with age, in a way that limbs and head compared with trunk is too short. The upper arm is especially short in the forearm, so that the finger cannot touch trochiter. Tibia and fibula are also short and disproportionate as compared to the femur and trunk. Therefore, while sitting the patient with short stature has the same height as a healthy person, but shorter when standing. This kind of patient has a difficulty in squatting, upright bending of the knees, and compensatory lumbar lordosis, has sudden, flat feet below he hip, and feet like a bear's paw. Patients walking is like duck step. A few patients can have intra-articular loose bodies, the so-called "joint mice". When "joint mouse" stuck in a joint, the joint twists.

5.4.3 How to Diagnose the KBD

5.4.3.1 The Clinical Diagnosis of KBD

KBD is a typical endemic disease. Endemic area contact history is strictly necessary condition. KBD severity is divided into degree I, II, III. Degree I is the enlargement of finger joints, Grade II is brachydactylia, and Degree III is short limb deformity (Fig 5.8-5.10). KBD progression is relatively slow. Most patients have no obvious symptoms in the early stage of onset. Some of the patients in the early onset feel weak, easy fatigue, muscle pain, formication of limbs, numbness, etc. The typical patient's joints are tight and the joint movement is not flexible, but after slight movement the syndrome can be relieved. Joint pain is the main symptom of most patients. In early stage of KBD, patients have fingers bent to the palm side slightly

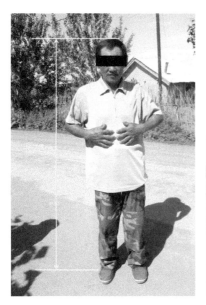
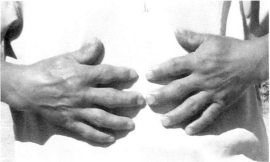

Fig. 5.8　KBD patient of Degree Ⅰ. At the early stage of the disease, there occurs symmetrical pathological enlargement of multiple finger-joints, or slight flection of elbow.

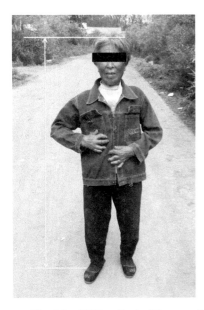

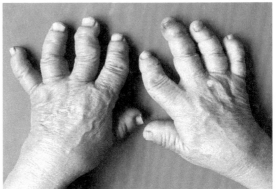

Fig. 5.9 KBD patient of Degree Ⅱ. Besides the changes of Degree Ⅰ, deformed short fingers or toes, and enlarged joints of wrists, knees and ankles can be observed. It is hard for KBD patients to crouch, and their gait resembles duck's walk.

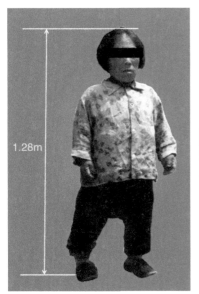

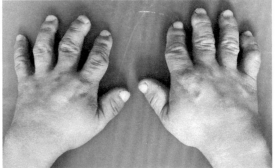

Fig. 5.10 KBD patient of Degree Ⅲ. Obviously short limbs, and dwarfism with normal intelligence is detected.

with fingertip goose-head-shaped drooping, joint thickening occurs in finger and toe joint, and gradually in the wrist, elbow, knee and ankle joints. Shoulder and hip joints can be affected in patients with advanced severe condition. Interphalangeal joint thickening of distal finger is like abacus beads; the back of fingertip may have a transverse ridge called Herb's tubercles. Patients with severe condition may have short finger or short limb deformity. Fingers, toes, wrist, elbow, knee, ankle joint can be seen dislocation or subluxation. The height of the patient is not commensurate with age, his head and limbs compared with his trunk unsymmetrical shortening. The upper arm is especially shorter than forearm.

5.4.3.2 The X-ray Images of KBD.

KBD is an osteoarthropathy with joint injury of limbs. The X-ray image of hand can reflect the degree of pathological lesions and the damage of the joints in the whole body, and there is no difference between the change of large joints, such as the elbow in KBD and that in OA. Therefore, we can regard the X-ray image of hand as the basis of diagnosis and differential diagnosis. In addition, characteristics of the KBD change with collapsed ankle talus and the shortened calcaneus, can be used for the diagnosis of atypical KBD.

The earliest pathological change of the patients with KBD is found in hand metacarpophalangeal, especially from the second to fourth maniphalanx. The pathological changes start from metaphysis, then expand to the epiphysis and carpal bone. The first changes are metaphyseal wavy or zigzag structure,and the upper bone trabeculaes of calcification zone also become unevenly thick. The second change is that temporary calcification zone is incomplete, depressed and hardened. The third changes are that articular surface of distal end of phalanx become depressed, incomplete, cystoid and defective, while epiphyses become deformed, lytic or broken, and early closure of metaphysis-epiphysis appear.

The changes of metacarpals are the same as that of the phalanges, but appear later than those of the phalanges. For carpal bones, damage of Os capitatum appears earlier, and the proximal end of Os capitatum has crescent-shaped defect. The development of disease can involve other carpal bone (scaphoid, lunate, triangular bone, trapezium, trapezoid bones, and hamate). The margin of carpal bone is irregular and sclerous, and small deformations and crowdings may be seen in the carpal bones of patients with severe conditions. The X-ray imaging features of advanced KBD include beak-shaped, coronary hyperplasia formation of bone spurs, bone ridge, bone spine and joint space narrowing. The mild cases only show proliferation at proximal and distal ends of first or second phalanx. Such cases are most likely due to childhood suffering from the metaphyseal bone or bone Mid-Mid-KBD. For the severe cases, the bottom of the phalanx becomes wide or flared bell-shaped, and articular surface is uneven with depression. The patient's fingers are not short, but crooked. Such cases are most likely to be suffering from childhood Mid-metaphyseal bone epiphysis KBD sequelae. In addition to the above image, the severe cases show seriously damaged distal phalanx, the stubby diaphysis and varus deformity, which are the continuation of pathological changes of children bone-joint-typed case.

5.4.3.3 Diagnosis and X-ray Image of Children KBD

The children KBD in early cases do not have the clinical signs. Even in the pandemic period, the ratio of early childhood cases developing into clinical cases does not exceed 50%. The diagnosis of children KBD relies on X-ray images. Children KBD X-ray radiographic signs of the fundamental change include mainly cysts, pseudocysts, metaphyseal irregularity, vertical spur formation of metaphyseal bone, metaphyseal widening sclerosis, metaphyseal depression, metaphyseal depression associated with sclerosis, bone end and joint surface defect, bone end Cutting angle sign, bone side spurs, bone-side cigarette-shaped sign, bone side depression, cone-shaped epiphyses, epiphysis deformation, line-shaped epiphysis, epiphyseal fracture, splayed epiphysis, epiphyseal delay (epiphysis dissolution, epiphyseal defect) and carpal edge sclerosis. There are one, two or more radiographic changes in the same case. At the same time, the radiographic changes must occur at multiple sites of more than one finger.So, changes at single site of single finger are not classified as KBD. The earliest changes start with metaphyses, and then advances to the bone-side or epiphysis. Especially the first and second phalanges of the index fingers, middle fingers or ring fingers are most likely involved. Based on the different lesions, KBD X-ray changes are divided into 6 types including metaphysis-type, metaphysic-epiphysis type, bony-end-type, bony-end-metaphysis-type, epiphysis-metaphysis-type and bone-joint-type (Fig. 5.11).

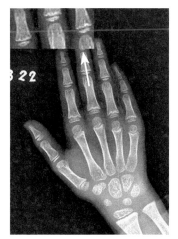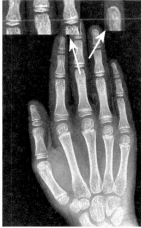

Fig. 5.11   8-year-old girl metaphysis type, index finger, middle finger, ring finger metaphyseal serrated, wavy change (left). 10-year-old girl metaphysis type, index finger, middle finger, ring finger metaphyseal irregular (right).

5.4.3.4   *Diagnosis and X-ray Images of Adult KBD*

Adult KBD patients are the sequelae of children KBD. Although there are some similarities between adult patients and child patients in X-ray imaging, there are clear differences. Therefore, recognising the basic X-ray signs of adult KBD are also very important. There are 10 basic signs of X-ray imaging changes, including pseudocyst, bone spine/bone crest/spurs, tuberositas hyperplasia and osteophyte, dissociative bone piece, defect or damage of articular surface, broadened base and spindle-like changes, bellbottom-like changes, collapse-restoration phase, metacarpal bone enlargement, subluxation and sickle shadow, carpal congestion and deformation, most of which coexist, constituting the characteristics of proliferation accompanying joint space narrowing for the KBD patients in degree I, as well as degree II and degree III (degree III is based on degree II and short stature) and characterized by brachydactylia.

5.4.4   What Is the Pattern of Joints Involvement in the KBD

KBD is a systemic disease, but the main lesions are bone joints, especially the limbs and joints. Disease has minor effects on the hands, wrists or feet, ankles, slightly heavier affected parts are elbows, knees, and might involve the shoulder, hip, spine and other joints. It has symmetrical multiple joint involvement, but the discreet side is more serious.

5.4.5　Why the Joints of KBD Patients Become Enlarged and Deformed

KBD mainly involves cartilage and bone, especially the bone of the limbs, shows degeneration and necrosis in hyaline cartilage with absorption of reparative changes. Chondrocytes are common in the coagulation necrosis, and the nuclei were fixed, and the cells were broken and dissolved. In the necrotic areas, there can also be further disintegration, liquefaction and necrosis foci in the presence of cartilage cells, which often show reactive hyperplasia, the formation of different size chondrocytes. In the adjacent bone tissues, the necrosis can occur as pathological calcification; the primary bone marrow blood vessels and connective tissue in the necrotic foci ossify, and eventually is replaced by bone tissue.

5.4.6　Why Some KBD Patients are Short statured

Cartilage lesion is the basic pathological change of KBD, necrosis of epiphyseal cartilage mainly occurs in the mast cell layer, even through the whole layer of epiphyseal plate. After deep necrosis in epiphyseal plate, as vessel from the metaphysis cannot invade, normal cartilage ossification activities cease; but survival chondrocyte proliferation layer above the necrotic foci can continue proliferation, differentiation, resulting in partial epiphyseal plate thickening. In the near edge of bone necrosis foci often occur degenerative calcification, and deposits along the metaphyseal bone necrosis edge forming irregular bone or transverse beam, forming irregular trabecular bone fragments or cross, indicating normal ossification process to a halt. While the rest osteoblast activity of epiphyseal plate continues, it results in epiphyseal ossification lines of uneven thickness and uneven. When the focal necrosis throughout the epiphyseal plate, necrosis absorption, organization and ossification are carried out by the two directions-epiphyseal and metaphysea, it finally leads to early bone epiphyseal plate closure, the longitudinal growth of the early bone stop, causing the short finger (toe) or Phocomelia, the formation of little sign fingers.

5. 4. 7　What is the Difference between KBD, Rheumatoidarthritis and Osteoarthritis

The basic pathological changes of rheumatoid arthritis are synovitis. There is a peripheral type, aged 25-40, child type occurring among children under 15 years old, and a mixed type of the clinical characteristics partly shared with the two previous ones. Its occurrence is more acute and combined with fever, occasionally rash and swollen lymph nodes, leukocytosis, joint swelling and exudation, as well as rheumatoid factor detected in laboratory tests at higher than normal level. Primary osteoarthritis, also known as degenerative joint disease, is a multiple chronic osteoarthritis, mostly scattering in the occurrence of multiple age in middle-aged. It appears earlier in large joints than small joints, with pain increasing significantly when patients exercise.

Traumatic osteoarthritis is mostly a scattered event, in which the patient has a history of trauma, and lesions may involve multiple sites or a single site, and all age groups can be attacked by it. Peel osteochondritis developing mainly from trauma, is common in athletes, and it often occurs in joints of the knee and ankle. The main symptoms are joint pain, joint twisting and loose bodies within the joint effusion.

KBD is an endemic disease whose onset age is 7-12 years old children and adolescents. The onset of small joints happens earlier than that of large joints. There is pain after rest, and there is not acute attack or obvious inflammatory reaction. Bone of the joint becomes thickened. Moreover, joint twisting and intra-articular loose body can occur in severe cases.

5. 5　Prevention and Control of KBD

Although the etiology of KBD is not clear, the KBD control strategy proposed by professor YANG Jianbo cuts off the chains of causation and blocked the ways that pathogenic agents enter the body, which made a successful progress in preventing and control KBD in China. In 2000, Disease Control Department of Chinese Ministry of Health had put the main suggestions of strategy in "Project planning for comprehensive prevention and control of key national endemic diseases (2001-2005)". In April 2003, Chinese strategy for control of Kashin-Beck Disease won first prize of medical science and technology progress prize of Heilongjiang Province. The strategy included 5 points, which are (1) To exploit paddy field instead of dry field and to consume rice as staple food in places where water resources is abundant; (2) In remote mountainous area, especially the western region, farmland should be returned to forest or grass; (3) To plant vegetables or economic crops and import cereal from non-KBD areas if transportations of KBD endemic areas are convenient or wards near the town or city; (4) If the KBD endemic areas do not have conditions that mentioned above, adopting measures as possible, such as scientific farming and dry storage, to reduce the content of T-2 toxin in the staple food (i.e. wheat flour and maize) below 100ng/g, at least less than 300ng/g; (5) "Relocation and Education" and "Centralized Schooling". At present, more than 95% of KBD areas have been implemented with comprehensive prevention and control measures, by which KBD has dropped to the lowest level in history.

5.5.1　Effects of Improved Grain Quality and Agricultural Methods on KBD

In the view of the theory that mycotoxins were the causative factor of KBD, a trial of changing grain to prevent KBD was put into practice, which gradually got obvious effect. After relevant experts made an examination and review on the effects of changing grain for prevention of KBD, as well as unified diagnostic criteria for KBD, they divided prevention and control of KBD in China into four periods. The first period refered to 1950s when the method of changing grain was the main prevention measure. In 1954, in Xichuan village of Fusong County in Jilin Province was the first village to adopt the method of changing grain for revention of KBD. In 1957, Wudian of Qianxian County in Shaanxi Province, the measure of changing grain was implemented. In 1958, in Shitouhezi of Shangzhi County in Heilongjiang province, the same measure was executed.

　　From 1960s to 1970s is the second period. Many kinds of methods of improving water quality, including digging deep wells, importing spring water, filtering water and adding sulfur, gypsum into drinking water, were widely carried out for the prevention and control of KBD. In December of 1979, a national symposium of improving drinking water for prevention and control of KBD was held in LinFen City of Shanxi Province. During the conference, the stage summary was made in view of various water-improving experiences from different places. During this period, KBD research laboratory of Harbin Medical University performed the test of changing grain to prevent KBD in Xincun, Baoshan Mining Area of Shuangyashan City. It took five years (from 1972 to 1977) to make the more than two thousand population of KBD village the first basically controlled experimental area.

The third period was 1980s. Central office of endemic disease confirmed that the method of changing grain had obvious effect on prevention and control of KBD. During 1979-1982, Central office of endemic diseases initiated and organized KBD scientific investigation in Yongshou. It performed the repeated verifications on the measure of supplementing selenium to prevent KBD, as well as gave a careful observation on the methods of changing grain and improving water for prevention of KBD. Thereafter, measures of supplementing selenium to prevent KBD were widely implemented in Gansu, Heilongjiang, Shaanxi, Henan, Hebei, Inner Mongolia and other provinces. In 1988, according to the endemic annual statistics, the number of people accepting measures of changing grain nationwide was nearly 1 million, the number of people accepting the measure of complementing selenium was 12.243 million, and the number of people accepting the measure of improving drinking water was nearly 20 million.

The fourth period was 1990s. In 1990s, through the practice of prevention and control and the further study on the cause of KBD, the theory of Chinese KBD prevention and control policy was formed. The main points are as below. (1) In KBD areas, if the condition of water source is allowed, dry farmland should be changed into paddy field and the staple food should be changed into rice; (2) In some KBD areas, where the transportation is convenient or which are near towns, the planting grain should be switched into planting vegetables or other economic crops, and staple food should be purchased from markets; (3) In the remote mountainous areas, returning farmland to forest or returning farmland to pasture is feasible; (4) In places, where the above conditions are not available, the planting grain scientifically, and keeping dry conditions for grain storing to reduce food pollution degree should be publicized.

In the late 1990s, Gross Domestic Product increased rapidly, and people's living standards were greatly improved. Children of KBD families in some KBD areas migrated to the boarding schools of non-KBD areas to acquire education, which was called "Relocation and Education". The government also implemented a poverty relief project for children in the poor areas of the western China,namely, small-scale primary and secondary schools in remote poor areas were merged into a large-scale school with good education conditions located in towns. Therefore, children of school age lived and studied in the school freely. This boarding school model was called "Centralized Schooling". Due to "Relocation and Education" and "Centralized Schooling", the children in KBD areas were separated from the KBD areas and ate staple food produced in non-KBD areas, which was equivalent to "relocation and changing grain". This appeared effective to prevent KBD.

　　Throughout the experiences for prevention and control of KBD during the four stages, researchers work on prevention and control of KBD summarized a comprehensive prevention and control measures, which meant "Returning Farmland to Forest or Returning Farmland to Pasture", "Changing Grain", "Relocation and Education" and "Centralized Schooling".

5.5.2　Effects of Selenium Supplementation on KBD

As Se deficiency is considered a main risk factor for the occurrence and development of KBD, various forms of Se supplements have been administered in most endemic areas since 1970's. The most common types of Se supplements in China are oral sodium selenite tablets (Se-tablet), Se-enriched salt, Se-enriched egg, Se-enriched tea, Se-enriched yeast, and combination therapies (e. g., vitamin E, iodine or zinc gluconate, and Se). Crop dusted with selenium, Se-enriched fertilizer, and some more comprehensive measures, such as improvements in water source and food quality, and improvements in general hygiene conditions have been also implemented.

5.5.2.1　Sodium Selenite Tablets

In the late 1970s, oral Se-tablet was adopted to treat KBD. Dosage was determined depending on patient's age. Usually, children under five were given 0.5 mg Se per week, five- to nine-year-old took 1 mg per week, and children older than nine took 2 mg per week. When a long-term observation experiment was conducted among children aged three to ten years, the X-ray detection rate of metaphysis of phalanges in KBD significantly decreased from 42.55% in 1976 to 4.09% in 1983. Among the children who had started the treatment before three years of age, none was contracted with KBD during this period. A series of clinical trials has proved that this method is effective in improving the membrane stability of chondrocytes, ameliorating the metaphyseal lesions, improving the Se nutritional status, promoting the repairing action of the lesions both in metaphyses and the distal end of phalanges in hands, and preventing its deterioration in hand of KBD children. Before the intervention, the mean hair Se content was lower than 100 ng/g; two years after accepting this treatment, it rose to 200 ng/g or even reached the level found in samples from the non-KBD area. A trial involving 420 children showed that no one was deteriorated in the intervention group with 81.9% of X-ray improvement rate, whereas in the control group, only 39.6% of subjects improved. Moreover, 13.19% of patients in control group had the aggravated symptoms.

5.5.2.2 Se-enriched Salt

Cooking salt containing sodium selenite (16.7 mg/kg) was introduced into the daily life of residents in KBD areas; the method achieved good results for prevention and treatment of KBD. Now, more than 1.03 million residents in Chinese KBD areas with low-Se nutrition are supplied with Se-enriched salt. In 1986, a comprehensive clinical trial presented results of a Se-enriched salt supplementation. At the baseline, average X-ray detection rates of metaphyseal lesions in the hands of KBD children were 57.1% in the Se supplement group (Se+group, supplemented with Se-enriched salt later) and 61.9% in the control group (Se-group, without Se supplement). Two and a half years later, average X-ray detection rates of metaphyseal lesions in Se-enriched salt supplementation group were decreased to 36.3%, but it was 45.4% in the non-Se-enriched salt supplementation group. Moreover, no new cases were detected in Se-enriched salt supplementation group, while 0.8% incidence was observed in the non-Se-enriched salt supplementation group. Eight months later, in Se-enriched salt supplementation group, the total rate of metaphyseal changes in phalanges was decreased from 45.65% to 9.10%, with no new case was reported. The severity of KBD was decreased as reflected by the high prevalence in KBD areas that dropped to mild level, or even the level close to those in non-KBD areas. However, in non-Se-enriched salt supplementation group, the incidence was 8.56%. Se-rich salt supplementation also substantially increased the Se nutritional status in vivo; the hair Se content of children from KBD area in Tibet rose from 74 ± 45 ng/g in 2001 to 256 ± 133 ng/g in 2003.

5.5.2.3 Selenium-fortified Wheat

The soil-food-body route is the major pathway from the environment to the human body. Se-fortified fertilizer and Se-fortified wheat (sodium selenite spraying on the leaf at 1g per 0.17 acre during wheat flowering stage) have been widely used in KBD areas. The Se content in Se-sprayed wheat increased to 75 ± 0.7 ng/g (17 ± 0.6 ng/g in the controls), while not differences of Fe, Mn, Mg, Ca, Mo, Sr, Cu and P contents were observed between the two groups. After consumption of Se-fortified wheat for 6 months, the Se content of children's hair and urine reached the level in samples from the non-KBD area (hair Se: 200 ng/g, urine Se: 5 μg/24 h).

During 1983-1988, a five-year trial verified the efficacy of Se-fortified wheat with Se-containing preparations. A significant negative correlation was discovered between Se content in whole blood/hair/urine and the X-ray detection rate of metaphyseal lesions of hands in children. At the base line, no significant difference was observed in the Se contents of whole blood between the Se supplemented group and the control group. However only half a year later, the Se content of whole blood in supplemented group quickly reached the level of 133 ± 27 ng/g, the X-ray detection rate of metaphyses in phalanges of children was declined from 58.76% to 46.15%, and the improvement in the rate of metaphyseal lesions reached 80.0%. Meanwhile, the Se content of whole blood in supplemented group was only 35 ± 15 ng/g, the X-ray detection rate of metaphyses in phalanges of children increased from 42.67% to 48.32%, and the improvement rate of metaphyseal lesions only 43.1%. Metabolically, in comparison with the levels before the Se-spray intervention, the level of urine creatinine significantly increased, while the urine creatine substantially decreased. The urinary hydroxyproline, ester sulfur, and inorganic sulfur showed an upward trend, while the urinary glycosaminoglycan levels changed with the season. The contents of urinary creatinine, urinary glycosaminoglycan, and the Se content of hair/urine were negatively correlated with the X-ray detection rate of metaphyseal lesions in hand of children.

5.6 The Treatment and Its Unified Evaluation Standard for KBD

5.6.1 How to Treat the KBD

KBD is a chronic, endemic, deformation osteoarthropathy. Its pathological characteristics are necrosis, degeneration, and degradation of articular cartilage and growth plate cartilage. The severe cases show short stature, disability and even loss of life skills. Clinically, the primary symptoms of KBD are joint pain, morning stiffness, enlarged and shortened fingers, and deformed and enlarged joints with limited motion in the extremities. Knee pain and functional limitations of KBD patients were reported as main factors affecting their daily life and ability to work well. Therefore, relieving knee pain and reducing functional disability are important for adult KBD patients.

The treatment of adult KBD is a significant clinical challenge. Currently, no KBD treatment guidelines exist in the literature. As the KBD patients share similar degradation of the cartilage matrix as osteoarthritis, but both have different etiologies. So, therapy of KBD is derived from experiences in osteoarthritis treatment. In accordance with the diagnosis standard for KBD (WS/T207-2010), the obvious joint pain and dysfunction of the adults KBD can be treated with non-drug therapy, medication or surgery, according to the seriousness of his illness (Table 5.2).

Table 5.2 Present Situation of KBD Therapy

Therapy	Description
1. Non-drug medication	Self-behavior therapy
	Operation support
	Acupuncture, massage and physical therapy
2. Drug medication	Prescription medicine (acetyl amino phenol, ibuprofen, meloxicam and celecoxib)
	Nutrition drugs (glucosamine sulfate, glucosamine hydrochloride)
	Injection administration (sodium hyaluronate)
	Chinese medicine (Jiangu Tablets)
3. Surgical treatment	Small incision free body excision
	Limited arthroscopic decompression bored and clean-up
	United arthroscopic clean-up add osteotomy
	Open joint clean-up or merger of osteotomy
	Artificial joint replacement

5.6.1.1 Non-drug Treatment

Non-drug treatment can be applicable to the KBD with mild joint pain and dysfunction, and can be used as auxiliary treatment in the process of drug and surgical treatment. It consists of three types of treatment. Firstly, self-behavior therapy: advocating walk right amount ground exercise, avoid unreasonable behavior of long time squats, climbing, running, jumping and sit on the ground damp. Secondly, operation support: cane, walker, and so on. Thirdly, acupuncture, massage and physical therapy: including heat, spas, Chinese medicine fumigation, electrotherapy, ultrasound, cupping, iontophoresis treatments and various physical therapy methods.

Acupuncture points and acupuncture technique based on ordinary institutions of higher education teaching material of "11th five-year plan" national planning "acupuncture" relevant section:for wrist choose Yang chi point, Yang gu point and Yang xi point; Knuckle selected Ba xie point; for elbow joint select Qu zhe point, Qu chi point and Chi zhe point; for knee joint select He ding point, Rou xi point and Wai xi point; and for ankle joint selected Jie xi point, Tai xi point and Kun lun point (Fig. 5.12, Fig.5.13).

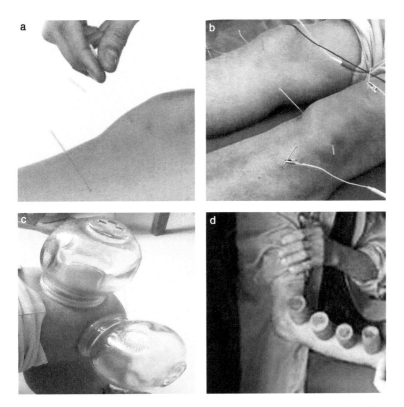

Fig. 5.12 Traditional Chinese Medicine, a-b: acupuncture; c-d: cupping therapy

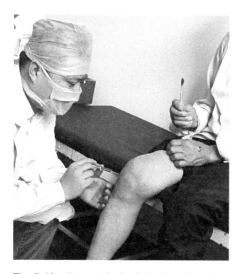

Fig. 5.13 Intra-articular injection of sodium hyaluronate is an effective treatment for intra-articular displaced fracture of the end of radius.

5.6.1.2 Drug Medication

The drug medication consists of the topical medications and oral medications. The topical medications are applied to the adult KBD mainly for elbow, knee, ankle joint pain and dysfunction. Topical medications can be various nonsteroidal anti-inflammatory analgesic drugs (NSAIDs), such as emulsion agent, paste, patches, and Chinese medicine, etc (Table 5.3). The oral medications are suitable for KBD with severe joint pain symptoms and joint dysfunction. Western medicine includes prescribed (ibuprofen, naproxen and celecoxib) and over-the-counter (acetaminophen and ibuprofen relievers) drugs, and cartilage nutrition (glucosamine hydrochloride, chondroitin sulfate), but hormonal drugs are strictly prohibited (Table 5.4). Recommend list of Chinese medicinal formulae according to the prescriptions.

Table 5.3   Recommend topical medications for KBD

Drugs	Dose	Times/day
Double chlorophenol acid diethylamine emulsion agent	Local	3-4
Ibuprofen emulsion agent	Local	3-4
Double chlorophenol acid patches	Local	1
piroxicam films	Local	1
Flurbiprofen Papua cream	Local	2

Table 5.4   Recommend oral medications for KBD

Drugs	Daily dose (mg)	Dose per (mg)	Time/Day	contraindication
Acetaminophen	2000 ~ 3000	300 ~ 600	3-4	severe liver and kidney function
Ibuprofen	1200 ~ 2400	400 ~ 600	3 ~ 4	

Continue

Drugs	Daily dose (mg)	Dose per (mg)	Time/Day	contraindication
Diclofenac sodium	75-150	25-50	2-3	
Miele Finn	100-200	100	2	severe heart function
Naproxen	500-1000	250-500	2	severe liver, kidney and kidney function
Loxoprofen	180	60	3	
Meloxicam	7.5-15	7.5-15	1	severe liver and kidney function
Celecoxib	200	100-200	1-2	sulfanilamide allergies
Glucosamine sulfate	720-1440	240-480	3	glucosamine sulfate allergies
Chondroitin sulfate	1200-2400	600-1200	2-3	

Note: NSAIDs are not recommended for pregnant women or nursing mothers, and persons with digestive ulcer bleeding/and allergies to aspirin.

5.6.2　Experience of Improving Joint Dysfunction of KBD Patient by Sodium Hyaluronate.

Sodium hyaluronate (SH), or hyaluronan, is assembled by alternating D-glucuronic acid and N-acetylglucosamine monosaccharides to form repeated disaccharides unit are linked into a linear straight-chain polymer, glycosaminoglycan sugar chain. Dr. Karl Meyer, professor of ophthalmology at Columbia University, firstly isolated it from bovine eye in 1934. SH is widely distributed in the joint cavity, blood vessels, eyes, heart, brain and skin. It shows a variety of important physiological functions in the body with its unique molecular structure and the physical and chemical properties. It lubricates joints, adjusts the permeability of blood vessel walls, regulates protein synthesis, diffusion and operating of the electrolyte to promote wound healing. SH in the synovial fluid is mainly synthesized by synovial membrane fibroblasts (Fig.5.14).

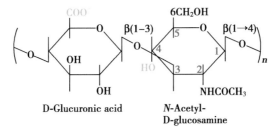

Fig. 5.14　Molecular structure of sodium hyaluronate

5.6.2.1 Physiological Function of SH

The physiological function of SH in patients with KBD is to promote the synthesis of endogenous hyaluronate, type II collagen and aggrecan in chondrocytes, cell proliferation and TNF alpha secretion, to enhance the expression of CD44, and to inhibit the action of the cartilage cell apoptosis. It can supplement joint synovial fluid levels of SH, improves the synovial fluid viscosity, rheological physical state and its motion. It can cover the surface of the articular cartilage and synovial membrane, repairs the damaged physiological barrier, prevents further loss of cartilage matrix and, thus, protect the articular cartilage. It is beneficial to the cartilage repair via lubrication of load-bearing articular cartilage surface, increasing the depth buffer elastic stress, and improving the activities of the joint function. It can provide chemical protective effect on articular cartilage by cutting down the level of prostaglandin in joint synovial fluid and limiting the spread of inflammatory mediators.

5.6.2.2 Treatment Method and Needing Attention

We recruited patients (over 18 years old) with KBD, who were capable of giving informed consent and had lived in the endemic areas for at least 6 months. Patients were eligible to participate in the study if they had a clinical or radiographic diagnosis of KBD in the knee. The clinical diagnosis of KBD was made by KBD experts at the institute of endemic diseases, health science center, Xi'an Jiaotong University according to clinical and radiological criteria (GB16003-1995). The patients were required to have been symptomatic for at least 3 months prior to enrolment. Patients were excluded based on the following criteria: (1) they had taken any medications for KBD during 3 months before enrollment; (2) they had a history or evidence of specified confounding disorders (e.g., septic arthritis, neoplasias, bone metabolic diseases, or osteoarthritis); (3) there were joint disorders such as joint fusion, deformity, cartilage damage severity, and articular cavity effusion; (4) they had allergies to poultry, feathers, or drugs; and (5) other patients who had serious adverse drug reactions had to be discontinued from the study. The treatment of KBD strictly followed the confirmed recommendations. SH was injected into the knee joint. Procedure included:(1) Patients with knee flexion 90° took a seat; (2) the knee skin was disinfected at patellar area and within the lower lateral approach; (3) the joint cavity was pierced in the direction of the medium and upward using the needle of # 7.5; (4) SH was injected after back to the suction without blood; (5) a sterile dressing was set after pull out of the needle; (6) patient's knee joint was bent several times after injection, to make sure that the drug is uniformly coated on surface of articular cartilage.

We strictly in performed the aseptic operation to prevent injection infection, and didn't wash the local after injection. Each injection was 2 ml, once a week, four to five weeks for a period of treatment.

5.6.2.3　*Therapeutic Effect of Intra-articular Hyaluronan*

Hyaluronic acid (HA) is one of the main components of articular cartilage and synovial fluid. Intra-articular hyaluronic acid (IAHA) has been widely employed in the medical management of knee osteoarthritis. Among the six meta-analyses and systematic-reviews performed to date, four trials gave positive conclusion that IAHA was an effective and safe treatment for osteoarthritis. Two trials had a small effect when compared with intra-articular placebo, which might have been overestimated due to publication bias. As adult KBD is a specific type of osteoarthritis, the clinical management of KBD may be educated by insights gained from the management of osteoarthritis. Thus, HA has been used to treat KBD, which showed that HA can markedly improve the function of the knee and relieve the symptoms of KBD.

One study was conducted to investigate the long-term efficacy and tolerability of hyaluronic acid in adult patients with KBD of the knee in four villages of Rangtang County, Sichuan Province, China. A total of 200 patients with KBD were examined; 67 patients (24.7%) failed the screening, and 113 patients were assigned and analyzed. Primary efficacy was assessed by a self-administered VAS score. Over 52 weeks, there was a reduction in knee pain as measured by the VAS pain scores. The VAS score was significantly reduced from 65.40 ± 12.10 mm (mean$\pm$SD) at baseline to 50.13 ± 12.05 mm ($P < 0.001$) after one injection (week 1) and continued to decrease until week 4. One week after the end of the active treatment phase, the VAS score was 35.39 ± 12.10 mm ($P < 0.001$). The treatment effect was sustained, and the

VAS score reached a minimum of 30.83 ± 12.01 mm at week 24, followed by a slight upswing in the VAS score at the end of the observation period (38.98 ± 12.76 mm, P <0.001 vs. baseline).

A meta-analysis of five trials on the overall effective rate, the pooled OR (95% CI) was 10.44 (3.57 ~ 30.51) favoring HA with the "fixed-effect" model. The effectiveness of the IAHA group and control group were 93.7% and 62.9% respectively, which indicated a significant difference in efficacy between the IAHA group and control group. After 2, 3, 6, and 12 months, the SMD (95% CI) for index of the knee joint was 0.95 (0.58-1.33), 1.47 (0.60-2.34), 1.25 (0.01-2.49) and 0.68 (0.51-0.84), the SMD in favor of IAHA ($Z = 1.97$-7.38, all P <0.05). Overall, the SMD (95% CI) in IAHA injection group was 0.79 (0.49-1.09). There was high statistical heterogeneity. The reduction of SMD for the index of the knee joint had been proved to be clinically effective.

5.6.2.4 Adverse Events

Five randomized controlled trials (RCTs) with a total of 848 intervention patients reported 26 cases of joint pain and swelling after injection, in which symptoms disappeared after 1 week without special treatment. One study mentioned two cases of joint effusion and one case of injection site bleeding. We did not count adverse reactions in the control group due to inconsistencies. Overall the rate of adverse events in IAHA groups was 3.1%.

5.6.3 Is the Surgery Effective for KBD Treatment

There is very little data on the safety and efficacy of treatments for KBD. Therefore, it is important to evaluate the curative effect and long-term efficacy of knee arthroscopic debridement in KBD patients. Here, one study showed that knee arthroscopy debridement had significantly improved the function of knee in KBD patients who had mild-to-moderate osteoarthritis over a long-term follow-up period. Therefore, this study suggested that arthroscopic debridement has long-term efficacy for KBD patients with Kellgren-Lawrence I-III classification. Another study reported data from 222 postoperative cases. They were followed-up for 1.5-5 years. There was no severe postoperative pain, dysfunction and prosthetic loosening, subsidence, tilt, dislocation, no deep venous thrombosis without pulmonary embolism, common peroneal nerve compression injury or complications, such as joint instability. Articular hematoma happened in two cases, and after aspiration of joint fluid the symptom disappeared. One case had superficial infection and recovered by the joint irrigation. The motor function of hip was evaluated by Harr hip score with excellent and good rate 72%.

Another study observed the limited clean-up arthroscopy plus drilling decompression in the treatment of knee with KBD. Eighty-six cases (100 knees) of patients with KBD were randomly divided into three groups: 1) a group of clean-up and limited arthroscopic drilling decompression, 2) another group of limited arthroscopic clean-up, and 3) the third group of arthroscopic drilling decompression. Followed up for 3 months to 1.5 years, Tegner knee evaluation comparison of knee joint function was carried out before and after treatment. After operation for 3 and 6 months, effective scores had no significant differences between limited arthroscopic clean-up group and limited arthroscopic clean-up and drilling decompression group. Two groups had significant difference from arthroscopic decompression drilling group. After operation for one and 1.5 years, the limited clean-up arthroscopy and drilling decompression group had significant difference from other groups. After operation for one and a half years, limited arthroscopic clean-up group had significant difference from arthroscopic decompression drilling group (Table 5.5). Conclusion was that the limited clean-up arthroscopy and drilling decompression treatment of knee with advanced KBD could relieve joint pain, improve joint function and the therapeutic effect.

Table 5.5 Comparison of scores of different periods in the different groups

Groups	Postoperative 3 months	Postoperative 6 months	Postoperative 12 months	Postoperative 18 months
A	9.85±1.04	8.32±1.67	7.73±0.94	6.03±1.24
B	9.24±1.43	8.26±1.76	5.82±0.41	4.35±0.74
C	7.36±0.98	6.03±0.85	5.34±1.03	2.98±1.31

Abbreviation: A group was clean-up and limited arthroscopic drilling decompression; B group was limited arthroscopic clean-up; C group was arthroscopic drilling decompression.

Patients with KBD scarcely have scientific knowledge in knee protection and exercise. Majority of KBD cases are from the endemic areas in rural China, where the population is largely poor with low socioeconomic indicators and low literacy. Therefore, health education and health promotion efforts are needed regarding conveying the importance of function exercises and put them into practice over extended periods of time. According to the different severity of disease, we consequently concluded that surgical treatment of adult KBD could alleviate the joint ache, improved joint function, and gave good and excellent outcomes.

5.6.4 Is There any Unified Evaluation Standard on Effect of KBD Treatment

Currently, there are hundreds of therapeutic effect scales and function evaluation criteria on osteoarthritis to evaluate benefits of drugs, surgery, rehabilitation, health education, and functional exercise. In summary, the criterion can be divided into two categories, which consist of medical assessment and questionnaire involving therapeutic effect and function evaluation. Evaluations of therapeutic effect have used different scores to investigate KBD. Ming Ling evaluated long-term efficacy of arthroscopic debridement on KBD using the Lysholm score. Chuan-tao Xia estimated hyaluronic acid and glucosamine sulfate for adult KBD using the Western Ontario and McMaster Universities Osteoarthritis (WOMAC) score and Lesquence score. Xin Tang's comparison of the efficacy and tolerability of hyaluronate acid and meloxicam in adult KBD used WOMAC score and VAS score, while Xin Tang's evaluation of total knee arthroplasty in elderly severe KBD patients was analyzed using VAS scores, Hospital for Special Surgery scores (HSS) and Functional Score. J. Yue comparison of chondroitin sulfate and/or glucosamine hydrochloride for KBD was performed using WOMAC score and SF-12. Rui Luo's comparison of efficacy of celecoxib, meloxicam and paracetamol in elderly KBD used WOMAC score. However, the Lysholm, WOMAC, Lesquesne, VAS, HSS, SF-12, and Functional Scores are all used for the evaluation of osteoarthritis scale (Table 5.6).

Table 5.6　The application of scale for KBD

Scale	Description
SF-36 (The MOS 36-Item Short-Form Health Survey)	It contains 8 dimensions of PF (Physical Functioning), RP (Role-Physical), BP (Bodily Pain), GH (General Health), VT (Vitality), SF (Social Functioning), RE (Role-Emotional) and MH (Mental Health) with 36 items.
SF-12 (The 12-Item Short-Form Health Survey)	It contains 8 dimensions of PF (Physical Functioning), RP (Role-Physical), BP (Bodily Pain), GH (General Health), VT (Vitality), SF (Social Functioning), RE (Role-Emotional) and MH (Mental Health) with 12 items.
EQ-5D(EuroQol-5 Dimensions)	the EuroQol Group coordinated a study that administered both the 3-level and 5-level versions of the EQ-5D included five dimensions of mobility, self care, usual activities, pain/discomfort and anxiety/depression.
WOMAC(The Western Ontario and McMaster Universities Osteoarthritis Index)	The Index is self-administered and assesses the three dimensions of pain, disability and joint stiffness in knee and hip osteoarthritis using a battery of 24 questions.
Lesquesne's index	It contains 6 content of joint rest pain, joint tenderness, swelling, movement pain, morning stiffness and the ability to walk with 11 items.
JOA (Japanese Orthopaedic Association Scores)	The JOA score has 4 parts of subjective symptoms, clinical signs, daily activities, and bladder function with 14 items, the total score of JOA is 29 and the lowest was 0.
Lysholm Scale	The scale consists 8 items of claudication, weight-bearing, interlocking, joint instability, pain, swelling, stair climbing, and squat.
WHO-DAS II (WHO Disability Assessment Schedule)	WHODAS 2.0 produces domain-specific scores for six different functioning domains-cognition, mobility, self-care, getting along, life activities (household and work) and participation.

Since the evaluation scoring of each study is not consistent, it is difficult to compare the differences of therapeutic effect, and how KBD in the clinical characteristics and severity are different from osteoarthritis. Therefore, the assessment instrument for therapeutic efficacy on KBD was developed relatively lately, when the Joint Dysfunction Index for therapeutic efficacy on KBD was released by Health and family planning commission. The KBDQOL (Quality of Life) is a simple and easy to use 28-item six-dimensional questionnaire, which includes body function, activity limitation, social support, economic, mental health, and general health. The measure has been developed as a true patient-based questionnaire and demonstrates good measurement properties. The KBDQOL questionnaire has demonstrated evidence of content validity, internal consistency, reliability, and construct validity, and it provides an objective tool for assessing quality of life of KBD. It can be used in clinical trials and observational studies to evaluate quality of life and intervention studies. As a KBD-specific instrument, it is likely to be a more sensitive and specific than the generic measures.

The Joint Dysfunction Index (JDI) of national health industry "Assessment for Therapeutic Efficacy on Kashin-Beck disease (WS/T 79-2011)" was released in 2011, which was used to evaluate the therapeutic effect of KBD. The JDI included five items: arthralgia during nocturnal rest (Q1), arthralgia on walking (Q2), morning stiffness (Q3), maximum walking distance (Q4), and activities of lower limb (Q5). Each item was divided into three grades (0 grade, 1 grade and 2 grade), with the total $0 \sim 10$ scores (Table 5.7). The calculation method for JDI was the following: the Sum of Joint Dysfunction Index (SJDI) = Q1+Q2+Q3+Q4+Q5. The improvement rate = [SJDI(pre-treatment)-SJDI(post-treatment)]/SJDI(pre-treatment) × 100%. Judging scale of therapeutic efficacy is as follows: if the improvement rate of SJDI is greater than or equal to 70%, it is judged to be markedly efficient; if the improvement rate of SJDI is greater than or equal to 30% and less than 70%, it was considered to be efficient. The improvement rate of SJDI less than 30% is considered to be non-efficient (Table 5.7).

Table 5.7   The Joint Dysfunction Index

Items	Grade	Score
Arthralgia during nocturnal rest	None	0
	Pain without affecting sleep	1
	Pain with affecting sleep, need to take drug	2
Arthralgia on walking	None	0
	Pain with more than 15min up/downhill (stairs) or walk	1
	Pain with less than 15min up/downhill (stairs) or walk	2

Continue

Items	Grade	Score
Morning stiffness	None	0
	Less than 15min morning stiffness of extremities joint	1
	More than 15min morning stiffness of extremities joint	2
Maximum distance walked	Walk more than 1000m	0
	Walk only 500-1000m	1
	Walk less than 1000m or in the bedroom and home	2
Activities of lower limb	Squats freely	0
	Squats difficulties or knee flexion less than 90 degrees	1
	No-squats or knee flexion more than 90 degrees	2

5. 7   More Experience of Prevention and Control of KBD

5. 7. 1   Experience on KBD Prevention and Treatment by Changing Grain in Shuangyashan Region

From 1972 to 1982, in Xincun brigade, Changsheng people's commune, Shuangyashan City the measure of changing grain for control of KBD had been implemented for ten years. From above studies two conclusions can be drawn. One is that, after changing grain during these years in Xincun brigade, the prevalence of KBD was obviously decreased and kept at a relatively consistent low level, which did not belong to the natural decrease resulting from the wave changes. Another is that the measure of changing grain is the only reason for control of KBD in Xincun brigade.

The main records of study included: (1) 1092 pieces of right-hand X-ray pictures taken from Grade 1-5 pupils in Xincun brigade during October of 1971 and August of 1974, (2) 768 pieces of right-hand X-ray pictures collected from Grade 1-5 pupils in Xincun brigade during August of 1974 and June of 1975, (3) 566 pieces of right-hand X-ray pictures from Grade 1-5 pupils from seven production brigades in Shuangyashan City during June of 1975 and July of 1975, (4) 325 pieces of right-hand X-ray pictures from Grade 1-5 pupils in Xincun brigade, Sixin second team and Lixin brigade during June of 1975 and July of 1975, and (5) General natural conditions and living conditions of the endemic area.

The KBD area on the outskirts of Shuangyashan City was Changsheng commune within a radius of 15 kilometers. Changsheng commune has nine production brigades with total population of about 5000 people.

The test of changing grain was carried out in Xincun brigade. In 1964, Xincun brigade was established to consist of 193 households of decentralized mine workers containing 1133 persons. The dwelling places of some commune members were in the middle of that of mine workers, while most commune members were living near the mine workers only one street away. The living conditions were basically identical, and the tap water was the only water source for miner workers and commune members.

At the beginning of the brigade's establishing (1964-1965), the commune members ate the same commodity grain as the mine workers did. In 1965 and 1966, the commune members ate half commodity grain and half self-produced grain. After the autumn of 1967, the commune members ate self-produced grain through the whole year. At the end of 1972, the brigade grew vegetables instead of planting grain. Commune members in the brigade mainly consumed commodity grain supplied by Baoshan grain shop, except for about 60 kilograms of self-produced grain gained from the brigade after 1972. The rest of the brigades in Changsheng commune kept consuming self-produced grain, and never changed to eat commodity grain, compared with Xincun brigade.

Shuangyashan KBD area was still an active area until 1980 (except for Xincun brigade which carried out changing grain). The main sign is that in the preschool children of most brigades the clinical detection rate of KBD was up to 40%, while X-ray detection rate was more than 60%, which was much higher than clinical detection rate. Among the children who had X-ray positive changes, the children who had metaphyseal change occupied a large proportion, up to 90%. According to these standards, the KBD area in Shuangyashan city is undoubtedly an active disease area, as shown in Table 5.8.

Table 5.8　KBD detection for grade 1-5 school children in 8 brigades
of Changsheng commune (1978)

Brigade name	Age group	Clinical detection rate (%)	X-ray detection rate (%)	Metaphyseal change in X-ray (%)
Tuanjie	6-17	37.0	62.2	98.0
Qingshan	7-16	72.3	80.6	100.0
Dongfeng	8-17	55.6	59.6	100.0
Hongwei	8-17	58.2	60.8	95.8
Fuqiang	6-18	52.7	83.5	76.1
Lixin	8-18	46.7	67.7	74.6
Sixin	10-15	49.5	66.4	82.5
Xincun	8-15	22.6	25.8	6.66

KBD was found in Xincun brigade in the winter of 1969. The disease development was so fast that inhabitants expressed their concerns strongly. In October of 1971, for the first time, an examination for diagnosis and an epidemiological investigation were performed in Xincun brigade. In the meanwhile, the children at the same age as those of the mine workers, who were living near the commune members and drunk the same water source with the commune members, got the same examination and investigation. The results are shown in Table 5.9. This kind of difference in Table 5. 9 is typical between the endemic area and non-endemic area.

Table 5.9　Comparison of KBD detection rates between children in Xincun
brigade and mine workers households

Population name	Detection number	Clinical detection rate (%)	X-ray detection rate (%)
Xincun brigade	125	44.0	75.8
Worker households	118	0.8	4.6

The distance between Xincun brigade and Lixin brigade is 7.5 kilometers. Both brigades were composed of decentralized mine workers. The time of the two brigades' establishment was basically similar, and the occurrence of KBD in both brigade was almost concurrent. The measure of changing grain was carried out in Xincun brigade, and the disease was controlled. On the contrary, in Lixin brigade, other measures, except for changing grain, were implemented, and the disease was still developing. Table 5.10 and Table 5.11 explain the characteristics of two brigades.

Table 5.10　X-ray detection for Grade 1-5 schoolchildren in Xincun brigade and Lixin brigade

Xincun brigade			Lixin brigade		
Detection time	X-ray detection rate (%)	Metaphyseal change in X-ray (%)	Detection time	X-ray detection rate (%)	Metaphyseal change in X-ray (%)
1971.10.	71.4	61.4	None	None	None
1974.03.	50.7	1.4	1974.08.	80.4	67.6
1974.12.	50.6	0.0	None	None	None
1975.06.	39.5	0.0	1975.07	82.3	74.8
1976.07.	31.6	3.2	1976.07	91.1	85.8
1977.10.	21.4	0.7	1977.06	86.5	80.2
1978.10.	25.8	1.7	1978.10	67.7	50.4

Table 5.11　New KBD case comparison between Xincun brigade and Lixin brigade

Location	Number of Grade 1-5 pupils with normal X-ray in 1974	Number of new KBD case from Grade1-5 pupils in 1975-1978	New incidence of KBD (%)
Xincun brigade	73	0	0.0
Lixin brigade	33	23	70.0

Sixi second brigade and Xincun brigade are about 1.5 kilometers apart. Since 1977, we began to recognize the special significance of Sixin second brigade, whose establishment time and population source were the same as that of Xincun brigade. The two brigades shared the single tap water pipe in daily life. Although KBD was controlled in Lixin brigade, KBD in Sixin second brigade kept developing, as shown in Table 5.12 and Table 5.13.

Xincun brigade and Sixin second brigade are in the same natural environment with the same water source, but KBD status in the two brigades was extraordinarily different. The prominent difference in various factors of living conditions was that Xincun brigade adopted the measure of changing grain, while Sixin second brigade did not do.

Table 5.12 Prevalence in children born in 1963-1970 in Xincun brigade
and Sixin second brigade

Location	Detection number	Clinical diagnosis rate (%)	X-ray detection rate (%)	Metaphyseal change in X-ray (%)
Xincun brigade	116	22.6	25.8	6.7
Sixin second brigade	24	62.5	62.5	66.7

Table 5. 13 Prevalence in children born in 1971-1975 in Xincun brigade
and Sixin second brigade

Location	Detection number	Clinical diagnosis rate (%)	X-ray detection rate (%)	Metaphyseal change in X-ray (%)	Epiphysis change in X-ray(%)	Distal end phalanx change in X-ray(%)
Xincun brigade	58	1.7	1.7	0	1.7%	0
Sixin second brigade	14	0	100	85.7	35.7%	64.3%

Above facts showed that the measure of changing grain received good effect for control of KBD. Since 1972, the staple food consumed by Xincun brigade was the same as that consumed by worker households, and basically no new KBD case occurred (Table 5. 14 and Table 5.15). Drinking water conditions among Sixin second brigade, Xincun brigade and worker households were identical, but staple food in Sixin second brigade was self-produced all the time and the incidence of KBD in Sixin second brigade stayed at high level, which suggested that consuming self-produced staple food was the key factor to cause KBD in Sixin second brigade.

Table 5. 14 Prevalence in children born during 1963-1971 (1978.11)

Location	Detection number	Clinical diagnosis rate (%)	X-ray detection rate (%)	Metaphyseal change in X-ray (%)
Xincun brigade	116	22.6	25.8	6.7
Sixin second brigade	24	62.5	74.2	66.7
worker households	85	0.0	4.7	0.0

Table 5.15　Prevalence in children born during 1971-1974 (1978.11)

Location	Detection number	Clinical diagnosis rate (%)	X ray detection rate (%)	Metaphyseal change in X-ray (%)
Xincun brigade	58	0.0	1.7	none
Sixin second brigade	14	0.0	100.0	85.7
Worker households	25	0.0	0.0	none

A few KBD cases occurred in worker households and Xincun brigade, which had implemented the measure of changing grain. After careful investigation, the answer was that those KBD patients ate self-produced staple food through various ways. For example, for worker households, some of them bought self-produced staple food from the KBD area, or some of them once visited and lived with the relatives in KBD area for a period of time. In Xincun brigade, a few of commune households consumed self-produced staple food for a while due to temporary financial trouble.

In summary, the experience for control of KBD in Xincun brigade of Shuangyashan city suggests that the fundamental reason that KBD gets controlled is to adopt the measure of changing grain.

5.7.2　Dietary Intervention Trial for the Prevention and Treatment of Children with KBD in Xinghai County and Guide County, Qinghai Province

5.7.2.1　Intervention Locations and the Choice of Intervention Objects

The trial for changing grain was divided into two stages. In the first stage of the trial, from August 2008 to September 2009, Xiemalang Village and Xinjianping Village in Guide County were chosen as intervention villages. The second stage of the trial is from September 2009 to October 2010, while Shang Village and Zhong Village of Tangnaihai Town in Xinghai County were selected as intervention villages. Children from 6 to 12 years old from the four villages were investigated with right-hand-X-ray examination. Based on these results, the children aged 6-11 were chosen as the intervention objects to monitor KBD.

5.7.2.2　Population Intervention Groups and Intervention Factors

As an epidemiological field investigation, based on similarity principle, i. e. the geographical environments, the diets, and the natural conditions were basically similar, the trial included two groups - control group and intervention group (grain-changing group). In the first stage, Xiemalang Village in Guide County was chosen as the grain-changing group, while Xinjianping Village in Guide County was chosen as the control group. In the second stage, Xia Village in Xinghai County was the grain-changing group and Zhong Village in Xinghai County was the control group. The children in the grain-changing group were given rice in terms of 150 kilograms per person per year and consumed rice per day (The rice was from Ningxia and T-2 toxin in the rice was 4.29 ng/g, far lower than that in the locally produced wheat and flour). The intervention was sustained for a period of one year, during which the children were visited to check the rice consumption every three months. The right-hand-X-ray examinations were performed every six months to determine the effectiveness of intervention measures.

5. 7. 2. 3 Quality Control

First of all, survey of baseline data must be accurate. KBD X-ray diagnosis must be made by three experts through double-blind method. Sample detection should be carried out complying with the quality standard of the laboratory. Prior to the implementation of intervention measures, the research group signed responsibility contracts with the Endemic Disease Institute of Qinghai Province, Center for Disease Control and Prevention (CDC) of Guide County and CDC of Xinghai County, supply and marketing stores and primary schools to ensure that the intervention measures were strictly put in place, as well as the regular observation and regular supervision were timely performed. The children and parents got knowledge of importance of eating rice to prevent KBD through popularization of health education for KBD. Parents ensured their children ate two meals of rice every day and schoolteachers checked the children's rice consumption every day. During the intervention period, the staff in CDC did follow-up every month, while the research personnel did visitation every three month.

5. 7. 2. 4 X-ray Examination Results before The Intervention Measure

In the first stage of the trial, 103 pieces of X-ray images were taken and 13 pieces of X-ray images were positive. Total X-ray detection rate was 12.6% with X-ray detection rate of 15.0% in Xiemalang Village and X-ray detection rate of 9.3% in

Xinjianping Village. In the second stage of the trial, 110 pieces of X-ray images were taken and 11 pieces was positive. Total X-ray detection rate was 10% with X-ray detection rate of 12.1% in Xia Village and X-ray detection rate of 6.8% in Zhong Village (Table 5.16).

Table 5.16   Children aged 6-12 X-ray detection in 4 villages of
Qinghai Province, 2008-2010

Location	Number	Number with me-taphyseal change	Number with Ep-iphysis change	Number for X-ray detection	X-ray detection rate (%)
Xinjiangping Village	43	2	2	4	9.3
Xiemalang Village	60	9	0	9	15
Zhong Village	44	3	0	3	6.8
Xia Village	66	8	0	8	12.1
Sum	213	22	2	24	11.3

5.7.2.5   Effect of Intervention Measures

(1) The detection rate of children's right-hand-X-ray

The intervention lasted for 1 year, during which X-ray examinations were conducted every 6 months. At the end of the first stage trial, X-ray detection rate of the control group rose to 9.68% from 6.45%, in the meanwhile, X-ray detection rate of grain-changing group dropped from 14.63% to 7.32%. At the end of second stage trial, X-ray detection rate of the control group rose to 32.26% from 6.06%, X-ray detection rate of grain-changing group rose to 13.46% from 11.76% (Table 5.17).

Table 5.17   Children aged 6-12 X-ray detection in Guide County and
Xinghai County of Qinghai Province, 2008-2010

Time	Group	Detection rate(%)		
		Before trial	Medium term of trial	At the end of trial
The first stage	Control	6.45(2/31)	16.13(5/31)	9.68(3/31)
	Grain-changing	14.63(6/41)	13.16(5/38)	7.32(3/41)
The second stage	Control	6.06(2/33)	12.90(4/31)	32.26(10/31)
	Grain-changing	13.46(7/52)	19.61(10/51)	11.76(6/51)

（2）New child cases of KBD and metaphyseal repair after 1 years of intervention

In the first stage of the trial, incidence rate of new children was 14.29% in the grain-changing group, which was significantly lower than that in control group (60%). Metaphyseal repair rate in grain-changing group was 57.14%, which was far higher than that in the control group (40%). Regarding the new incidence rate, it was lower in the grain-changing group than that in the control group by nearly 46%. In the second stage of the trial, the new incidence rate in the grain-changing group was lower than that in the control group by nearly 34%. In the grain-changing group, metaphyseal repair rate was 53.85%, which was significantly higher than that of control group. Therefore, the measure of changing grain was effective in preventing and treating the children with KBD (Table 5.18).

Table 5.18 New children case of KBD and metaphyseal repair after 1 years of intervention, 2008-2010

Time	Group	Total cases	New cases	New incidence (%)	Cases repaired	Repair rate (%)
The first stage	Control	5	3	60.00	2	40.00
	Grain-changing	7	1	14.29	4	57.14
The second stage	Control	10	8	80.00	0	0
	Grain-changing	13	6	46.15	7	53.85%

5.7.2.6 Conclusions

This trial was based on the historical data.Based on the hypothesis that the cause of KBD is mycotoxin-contaminating grain, intervention of changing grain was performed in considerably active KBD areas of Guide County and Xinghai County of Qinghai Province. Two stages of the intervention trial were carried out and main conclusions are as follows.

(1) Effect of changing grain to prevent children from KBD is significant. The children's X-ray detection rate in grain-changing groupclearly dropped, and the new incidence rate was lower than that in the control group, while the metaphyseal repair

rate higher than that in the control group.

(2) So far, changing grain is the safest and most economic measure to protect children from KBD.

Further Reading

1. A.V. Voshchenko, V.N. Ivanov. Kashin-Beck disease in the USSR. In: Proceedings of international workshop on Kashin-Beck disease and non-communicable diseases. World Health Organization. 1990;152-196.

2. Allander E. Kashin-Beck disease. An analysis of research and public health activities based on a bibliography 1849-1992. 1994, Scand J Rheumatol Suppl,99:1-36.

3. Takamori Tokio. Kaschin-Beck disease. Dysostosis enchondralis endemica. Japan. 1968.1:188.

4. Sokoloff L. Kashin-Beck Disease: Historical and pathological perspective. AIN Symposium Proceeding, American Institute of Nutrition Annual Meeting, (Washington DC), 1987:pp 61-63.

5. Yasuyuki Egashira. An outline of history of research on Kashin-Beck disease in Japan. In: Proceedings of international workshop on Kashin-Beck disease and non-communicable diseases. World Health Organization. 1990;149-151.

6. Sokoloff L. Acquired chondronecrosis. Ann-Rheum-Dis. 1990; 49(4): 262-264.

7. Ministry of Health in PR of China. Diagnosis of Kashin-Beck disease Ws/T207-2010. http:/www. moh.gov.cn/zwgkzt/s9500/201006/47920/files/810f8a8b47cf434195a59c071a97bdc0.pdf.

8. Ying Peipu. The clinical examination and diagnosis of Kashin-Beck Disease, edited by Ying Peipu. Scientific Publish House, Xi'an, 1987; pp1-99.

9. Guo Xiong. Diagnostic, clinical and radiological characteristics of Kashin-Beck disease in Shaanxi Province, PR China. International Orthopaedics (SICOT). 2001;25:147-150.

10. Tan Jian'an. The atlas of endemic diseases and their environments in the Peoples Republic of China. 1989; Beijing:Science Press, China.

11. Guo Xiong, Ding Dexiu, Zeng Lingxia, et al. The prospective study of relationship between low selenium and Kashin-Beck Disease. J XI' AN UNIV, 1999;11(1):1-7.

12. Mo Dongxu. Pathology of selenium deficiency in Kashin-Beck disease. In: Selenium in Biology and Medicine. Combs Jr.GF, Spallhoz JE, Levander OA, Oldfied JE, (New York) No strand Reinhold Company.1986,859-986.

13. Mo Dongxu, Ding Dexiu, Wang Zhilun, et al. Study on relationship between selenium and

Kashin-Beck disease in 20 years. Chinese J Control Endem Dis, 1997; 12 (1):18-21.

14. Guo Xiong, Zhang Shiyuan, Mo Dongxu. The role of low selenium in occurence of Kashin-Beck Disese. J X I'AN M ED UN IV (S), 1992, 4 (2) ：99-108.

15. Mo, D. X., Lv, S. M. Bai, C.. Progress of the relationship between low selenium and Kashin-Beck disease. Chinese Journal of Control of Endemic Diseases.1997; 9, 199-121.

16. Tan, J. A., Zhu, W. Y., Li, R. B., Zheng, D. X., Hou, S. F., Zhu, Z. Y. and Wang, W. Y.. Geographic distribution of Kashin-Beck disease in China and the relation of ecological chemico-geography to its occurrence. In: Proceedings of International Workshop on Kashin-Beck Disease and Non-Communicable Diseases. 1990; Chinese Academy of Preventive Medicine (CAPM). World Health Organization, Beijing, pp. 12-15.

17. Li, C. Z., Huang, J. R., Wang, W. L., Zhang, Y. X., Xu, J. M. and Wang, L..The experimental use of Se-diacetic acid in the prophylaxis and treatment of Kashin-Beck disease. Endemic Diseases Bulletin. 1988; 3, 81-83.

18. Liang, S. T., Mu, X. Z. and Zhang, F. J.. The observation on the effects of Kashin-Beck disease prevention by selenium salt. Journal of Practical Endemiology.1986; 1, 21-23.

19. Guo X, Ning YJ, Wang X. Selenium and Kashin-Beck disease. In: Selenium, Chemistry, Analysis, Function and Effect. 2015; Royal Society of Chemistry. London, pp.564-565.

20. Wang, D. S., Zhu, Z. Y., Luo, J. F.. The observation on the treatment of Kashin-Beck disease with sodium selenite and vitamin E. Chinese Journal of Endemiology. 1983; 2, 204-207.

21. Zhai Shusheng. Investigation on the relationship between Kashin-Beck disease and drinking water. In: Proceedings of international workshop on Kashin-Beck disease and non-communicable diseases. World Health Organization. 1990;96-101.

22. La Grange M, Mathieu F, Begaux F, Suetens C, Durand MC. Kashin-Beck disease and drinking water in Central Tibet. Int Orthop, 2001, 25(3):167-169.

23. Sun SQ; Zhao SJ; Liu ZhQ. The Correlation Analysis Between the Typical Ward of Kacshin-Beck Disease and Drinking Water in Western Sichuan Plateau. Earth and Environment, 2011, 39 (3): 363-370.

24. Peng A, Wang WH, Wang CX, Wang ZJ, Rui HF, Wang WZ, Yang ZW. The role of humic substances in drinking water in Kashin-Beck disease in China. Environ Health Perspect, 1999,107 (4):293-6.

25. Lei R, Jiang N, Zhang Q, Hu S, Dennis BS, He S, Guo X. Prevalence of Selenium, T-2 Toxin, and Deoxynivalenol in Kashin-Beck Disease Areas in Qinghai Province, Northwest China. Biol Trace Elem Res, 2015, [Epub ahead of print].

26. Zhang Y, Guo X, Ping Z, Yu M, Shi X, Lv A, Wang F, Wang Z. Main source of drinking water and familial aggregation of Kashin-Beck disease: a population based on case-control family study. Ann Epidemiol, 2009,19(8):560-566.

27. Sun LY, Li Q, Meng FG, Fu Y, Zhao ZJ, Wang LH. T-2 toxin contamination in grains and selenium concentration in drinking water and grains in Kaschin-Beck disease endemic areas of Qinghai Province. Biol Trace Elem Res, 2012,150(1-3):371-375.

28. Wang WZ, Guo X, Duan C, Ma WJ, Zhang YG, Xu P, Gao ZQ, Wang ZF, Yan H, Zhang YF, et al. Comparative analysis of gene expression profiles between the normal human cartilage and the one with endemic osteoarthritis. Osteoarthritis and cartilage/OARS, Osteoarthritis Research Society 2009, 17(1):83-90.

29. Wang S, Guo X, Wu XM, Lammi MJ. Genome-wide gene expression analysis suggests an important role of suppressed immunity in pathogenesis of Kashin-Beck disease. PloS one 2012, 7 (1):e28439.

30. Zhang F, Guo X, Wang W, Yan H, Li C. Genome-wide gene expression analysis suggests an important role of hypoxia in the pathogenesis of endemic osteochondropathy Kashin-Beck disease. PloS one 2011, 6(7):e22983.

31. Wang S, Guo X, Tan WH, Geng D, Deng BP, Wang CE, Qu X. Detection of serum proteomic changes and discovery of serum biomarkers for Kashin-Beck disease using surface-enhanced laser desorption ionization mass spectrometry (SELDI-TOF MS). Journal of bone and mineral metabolism 2008, 26(4):385-393.

32. Ma WJ, Guo X, Liu JT, Liu RY, Hu JW, Sun AG, Yu YX, Lammi MJ. Proteomic changes in articular cartilage of human endemic osteoarthritis in China. Proteomics 2011, 11(14):2881-2890.

33. HY Bi, ZL Wang, JH Chen, H Zuo, XW Tan, D Geng. A pathomorphological observation on blood cells in peripheral bloods and bone marrow aspirates of the children with Kaschin - Beck disease. Chinese Journal of Control of EndemicDiseases. 2001, 16(5):266-269.

34. Lu AL, Guo X, Aisha MM, Shi XW, Zhang Y, Zhang YY. Kashin-Beck disease and Sayiwak disease in China: prevalence and a comparison of the clinical manifestations, familial aggregation, and heritability. Bone 2011, 48(2):347-353.

35. Shi XW, Guo X, Lv AL, Kang L, Zhou YL, Zhang YZ, Wu XM, Bai YD. Heritability estimates and linkage analysis of 23 short tandem repeat loci on chromosomes 2, 11, and 12 in an endemic osteochondropathy in China. Scandinavian journal of rheumatology 2010, 39(3):259-265.

36. Guo X, Ma WJ, Zhang F, et al. Recent advances in the research of an endemic osteochondropathy in China: Kashin-Beck disease. Osteoarthritis Cartilage. 2014;22(11):1774-83.

37. Zhao Zhi-jun, Xu Xiao-qing, LI Qing. Present Situation of Kashin-Beck Disease Therapy. Medical Recapitulate. 2015,21(1):81-84.

38. Yue J, Yang M, Yi S, et al. Chondroitin sulfate and/or glucosamine hydrochloride for Kashin-Beck disease: a cluster-randomized, placebo-controlled study. Osteoarthritis Cartilage, 2012, 20 (7): 622-629.

39. Tang X, Zhou ZK, Liu G, et al. The long-term efficacy and tolerability of hyaluronic acid in adult patients with Kashin-Beck disease of the knee. Clin Rheumatol. 2015;34(1):151-156.

40. Yu FF, Xia CT, Fang H, et al. Evaluation of the therapeutic effect of treatment with intra-articular hyaluronic acid in knees for Kashin-Beck disease: a meta-analysis. Osteoarthritis Cartilage. 2014; 22(6):718-725.

41. Ling M, Sun Z, Yi Z, et al. Long-Term Efficacy of Arthroscopic Debridement on Knee Osteoarthritis in Patients with Kashin-Beck Disease. Cell Biochem Biophys. 2015 Feb 22.

42. Fang H, Guo X, Farooq U, et al. Development and validation of a quality of life instrument for Kashin-Beck disease: an endemic osteoarthritis in China. Osteoarthritis Cartilage,2012, 20(7): 630-637.

43. Shuangyashan sanitation and antiepidemic station, Department of Kaschin-beck disease of Harbin Medical University. The condition of Kaschin-beck disease prevented from spreading by change of grain in Shuangyashan endemic area is analysed with epidemiologic method. Chinese Journal of Endemiology. 1982, 1(1): 51-55.

44. Yang Jianbo. Mycotoxins and human diseases. Chinese Journal of Endemiology. Chinese Journal of Endemiology. 2002, 21(4): 314-317.

45. Yang Jianbo. Study on Chinese strategy for Kaschin-Back disease control. Chinese Journal of Endemiology. 1997, 16(3): 129-131.

46. Yang Jianbo. Epidemiological investigation report of Kaschin-Beck disease in Soviet Chita. Chinese Journal of Endemiology. 1991, 10(4): 226-228.

47. Yang Jianbo. Observation on effect of changing grain for KBD prevention in Qianxian County, Fusong County and Shuangyashan—historical review and observation for changing grain to prevent KBD. Chinese Journal of Endemiology. 1988, 7(4): 230-233.

48. Yang Jianbo. Continued annotation on "Chinese strategy for control of Kaschin-beck disease". Chinese Journal of Endemiology. 2004, 23(1): 3-6.

49. Yang Jianbo. Epidemiologic observation on the conditional changes and preventive effects for the Kaschin-Beck disease. Chinese Journal of Endemiology. 2003, 22(6): 512-516.

50. Tibet Kaschin-Beck Disease Study Group of China research center for endemic disease control.

Investigative report on the prevalence condition of Kaschin-Beck Disease (KBD) in Tibet. Chinese Journal of Endemiology. 2000, 19(1): 41-43.

51. Yang Jianbo. Research progress of Kashin Beck disease caused by Fusarium toxin. Chinese Journal of Endemiology. 1994, 13(2): 114-117.

52. Yang Jianbo. Report on the route of transmission of causative factor leading to Kaschin Beck disease. Chinese Journal of Endemiology. 1989, 8(6): 382-385.

Chapter 6

Keshan Disease

Shuqiu Sun, Hongqi Feng, and Jie Hou

Abstract

Keshan disease (KD) is a novel cardiomyopathy of unclear cause only occurred in some poor rural areas of China, characterized by obvious yearly and seasonal prevalence as well as vulnerability for self-sufficient farming population, killing hundreds of thousands of people over last century. Based on time course of onset and cardiac function of a suffering patient, KD is generally classified into four transformable types: acute type, sub-acute type, chronic type, and latent type. And their major clinical manifestations are cardiac dysfunction and arrhythmia.

KD was first recognized in medicine in the period of Japan invaded Northeast China. Since 1949, Chinese governments have made great efforts in fighting against KD epidemics, through broad social mobilization and engagement of local residents, especially deployment of substantial resources including money and medical teams to stem the outbreaks and save lives with combined measures. In 1960s, Chinese investigators achieved multiple groundbreaking discoveries in the control and prevention of KD -- several plausible etiological hypotheses, and highly effective approaches for emergency rescue of critically ill patients by high-dose intravenous vitamin C therapy, and for community-based primary prevention by selenium supplementation or balanced diet. Most importantly, since China's open policy in 1978, the overall prevalence of KD has begun to decline dramatically thanks to rapid economic development in affected villages, reaching the lowest level ever and sustaining a steady state. Ultimately, we won the battle, but at immense cost. Relevant sectors of governments have moved on, shifted from 1990 to focus on the disease surveillance and home care for heart failure, and believed that it would be completely eliminated following the implementation of poverty relief programs.

In this chapter, we provide basic knowledge on KD from perspectives of clinical medicine, pathology and epidemiology, and will particularly give emphasis on the major accomplishments and experiences worth spreading by reviewing its past control history.

6.1 The Discovery of KD

In the late fall of 1935, a terrifying epidemic of unknown origin hit several villages around Keshan County, Heilongjiang Province, leaving dozens of people dead within a month. Faced with this fatal disease, health authorities dealt with contact tracing and isolation completely in accordance with the control procedure for Plague, but shortly dismissed the stringent limitation because that no contagious effect was observed between individuals. And so, in the early 1937, they called it "Keshan disease" -- named after the first discovery place.

In fact, this condition had appeared as early as in 1907 according to an annal of Keshan County. On the other hand, a couple of records also found elsewhere: one stated that an epidemic of unknown origin occurred in 1911 in pear-tree ditch of

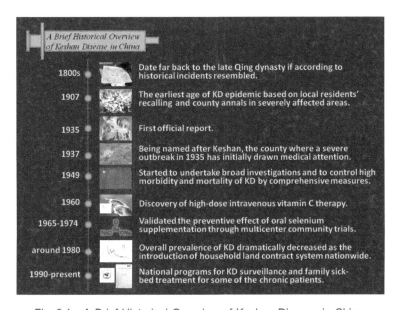

A Brief Historical Overview of Keshan Disease in China	
1800s	Date far back to the late Qing dynasty if according to historical incidents resembled.
1907	The earliest age of KD epidemic based on local residents' recalling and county annals in severely affected areas.
1935	First official report.
1937	Being named after Keshan, the county where a severe outbreak in 1935 has initially drawn medical attention.
1949	Started to undertake broad investigations and to control high morbidity and mortality of KD by comprehensive measures.
1960	Discovery of high-dose intravenous vitamin C therapy.
1965-1974	Validated the preventive effect of oral selenium supplementation through multicenter community trials.
around 1980	Overall prevalence of KD dramatically decreased as the introduction of household land contract system nationwide.
1990-present	National programs for KD surveillance and family sick-bed treatment for some of the chronic patients.

Fig. 6.1　A Brief Historical Overview of Keshan Disease in China.

Houhe village, Yanji municipality of Jilin province, which extremely assembled the description of KD clinical manifestations according to a medical official's survey report. The second record was seen in the inscription carved in a stone stood in Jinling Temple, Huanglong County, Shaanxi Province, reading that a disease called Yellow-Water Vomiting Disorder (YWV) assembling KD had prevailed there since 1858. So, it is hard to make clear the earliest date of KD occurrence. Historically, KD has been prevalent like surging waves over 100 years, threatening the life of local residents (Fig. 6.1).

6.2   Epidemiology

6.2.1   What's the Scope of Areas Affected by KD

KD occurred only in rural areas, and was distributed in a wide cold-humid and selenium-deficient zone from the northeast to the southwest, covering 25,768 villages of 328 counties of 16 provinces in middle of China. At township level, the population at risk is about 68.4 million.

Residence altitude of the patients with KD usually ranged from 100m to 2500m, extremely reaching 3000m. The area types of KD prevalence were diverse, including Da Hinggan and Xiao Hinggan Mountains, Changbai Mountain, Yanshan Mountain, Northwest Loess Plateau, Yunnan-Guizhou Plateau, Tibetan Plateau, Liangshan Mountain in Sichuan Dabashan, Hengduan Mountains in Yunnan province. The typical areas are northeast plain; southwest hills; and northwest loess plateau (Fig. 6.2).

6.2.2   Who are Susceptible to KD

Among the residents living in the endemic areas of KD, women of childbearing age and children aged 3-7 were the most affected; family aggregation was commonly seen in poor families, and these families were often the most socio-economically disadvantaged in the endemic areas, especially those who newly immigrated to the endemic areas.

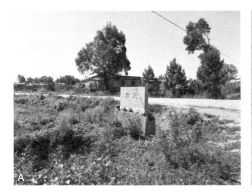
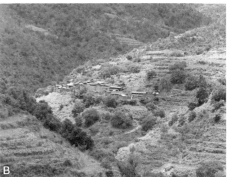
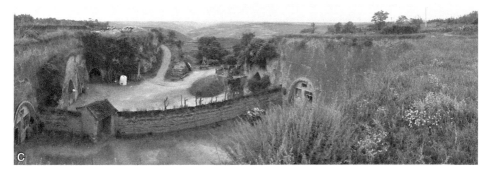

Fig. 6. 2   Natural landscape of typical villages affected by Keshan disease

6. 2. 3   Which is the Most Prevalent Month of a Year for KD

Despite being a non-communicable disease, KD is always liable to occur during some months of a year. The epidemic season varies in different regions of KD. In northern China, the prevalence peak for most acute KD patients lasts about 5 months from November to next March. The most typical areas of KD are in northeast China, including Heilongjiang, Jilin and Liaoning Province. While such provinces as Shandong, Shaanxi and Gansu are similar to northern China but not typical. However, the epidemic peak is completely opposite in southern areas, with morbidity of KD higher from June to October (Fig. 6.3). The pattern of KD patients is largely sub-acute.

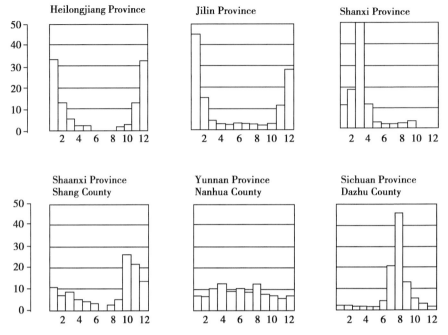

Fig. 6.3　Comparison of monthly morbidity of acute Keshan disease in different types of affected areas.

6.2.4　Is the Prevalence of KD Increasing or Decreasing

The prevalence of KD has been steadily decreasing since the late 1970s when China started economic reform. In 1964, the incidence of KD was 223 per ten thousand people in Fanrong Commune of Fuyu County of Heilongjiang Province. From 1969 to 1971, the incidence of Ganquan County in Shaanxi Province was 54-64 per ten thousand people. In 1966, the incidence in Dazhu County in Sichuan Province was 39 per ten thousand people. Since the late 1970s, KD incidence has dropped significantly (Fig. 6.4). Since 1990, no case of acute KD had been seen at the 24 national surveillance sites in 15 provinces. During 2000-2007, the prevalence of chronic KD was about 70 per ten thousand people, and the prevalence of latent KD was around 320 per ten thousand people in the 24 national surveillance sites in 15 provinces. The results of the national prevalence study of KD, conducted in 2008 (Fig. 6.5), showed that the prevalence of chronic and latent KD were 50 per ten thousand people, and 170 per ten thousand people, respectively. During 2009-2014, the preliminary results of the national KD surveillance were similar.

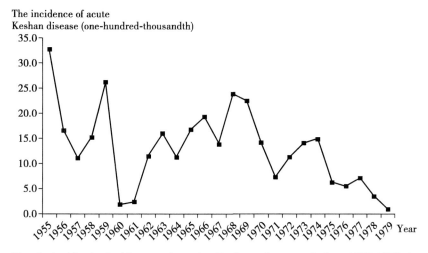

Fig. 6.4 Yearly incidence of acute Keshan disease during 1955-1979 in Northern China

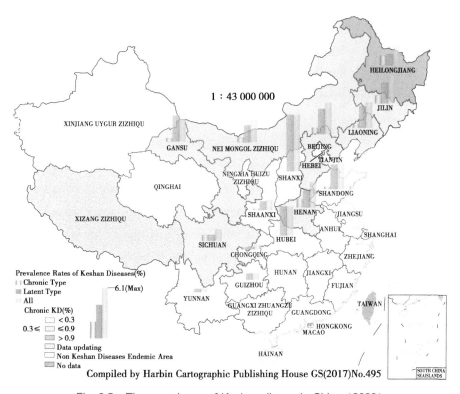

Fig. 6.5 The prevalence of Keshan diseae in China（2008）

217

6.3   Etiology

6.3.1   What's the Cause of KD

Plenty of etiologic investigations had been carried out since 1935, but the cause of KD remains unclear except for several plausible hypotheses including chronic carbon monoxide intoxication, dietary malnutrition, enterovirus infection, and longer consumption of mycotoxin-contaminated cereals. In 1960s, etiological studies of KD had led to a big controversy over either soil chemical origin, or biological origin. Most scientists believe that multiple factors in combination cause KD occurrence due to the imperfection of every single theory proposed. However, growing body of evidence from epidemiologic surveys suggested that locally planted cereals maybe the sole source of toxic agents for triggering KD.

6.3.2   Which Trace Element is Believed to be the Fundamental Risk Factor of KD

In the early 1960s, Xie et al proposed the hypothesis of soil and water origin, explaining migration of some chemical elements in soil and water may result in the loss of essential elements in cereals through food chain. In 1965, inspired by white muscle disease in cattle and sheep in KD affected villages, Guanglu Xu, observed that selenium could prevent the occurrence of KD using randomized controlled trial. In the mid 1960s, trials of KD prevention by oral administration of sodium selenite began in Shaanxi and Heilongjiang. In the 1970s, incidence of sub-acute KD was observed significantly lower than that of control group in Mianning County in Sichuan Province, and later in Xichang in the same province. It confirmed that selenium supplements could effectively prevent acute and sub-acute KD. In 1970, a team of geologists led by Tan et al found that low selenium in soil, water environments and the head hairs, nails and blood of the residents living in the endemic areas of KD was consistent with the regional distribution of KD from the northeast to the southwest in China. In addition, more results of epidemiological surveys showed reduced selenium content and activities of selenium-containing enzymes in local resident body, as well as lower selenium level in their soil, water and food compared with that from non-endemic areas. KD incidence shows a statistically significant negative correlation with blood selenium level. Subsequently, interventions by supplementing selenium to prevent KD were widely taken across the endemic areas in China, and achieved ideal results. Therefore, the selenium deficiency was widely recognized as the fundamental risk of KD. Weihan Yu even proposed "selenium deficiency plus unknown factor" as the etiological model for KD.

Some principle investigators were awarded the National Scientific Conference Prize in 1978, and the Krauss-Schwartz prize of the Society of Biological Inorganic Chemistry in 1984 for their discovery of selenium role in KD.

6. 3. 3   What's the Association of Enterovirus Infection with KD

The theory of viral infection proposed by Lin in 1961 based on more than 50 strains of viruses, e.g. Coxsackie virus, Echo virus, adenovirus and some undentified strains were isolated in the samples of the blood, autopsy myocardia and other materials of the patients with acute and sub-acute KD. Later in the 1990s, RNA fragments of enterovirus were detected in the myocardial specimens of patients with sub-acute and chronic KD by the techniques of in situ hybridization, polymerase chain reaction and monoclonal antibody. In serology, the neutralizing antibody titer of CVB1-6 was two times higher in the serum of patients with acute or sub-acute KD, and CVB neutralizing antibody titer was significantly higher in the sera of patients with KD than that of men, and some patients showed 4-fold increase. Detected virus-specific IgM antibody positive results were as high as 33-66.6%, indicating new CVB infection in KD patients. However, virus hypothesis is lack of evidence derived from trials.

6. 3. 4   What's the Association of Long-term Consumption of Moldy Grains with KD's Occurrence

Starting from 1957, the Institute of Epidemiology and Microbiology at Chinese Academy of Medical Sciences, and Heilongjiang Provincial Institute of Endemic Disease collaborated closely to investigate the underlying cause of KD. They found that there was always a contradictory phenomenon between biological origin view from epidemiological observations, and toxicosis view from clinical and histopathological manifestations, and suggested that an integration of various phenotypes of KD must be considered in etiologic studies. In August 1961, Guo et al proposed etiologic possibility of chronically consuming local cereals contaminated by mycotoxin based on the combined results from their field surveys, laboratory tests, and exchange trial of dietary grains. This hypothesis is the most promising theory in guiding the discovery of KD cause.

Later, Moniliformin, T-2 toxin, and citreoviridin were successively investigated the association with KD occurrence, unfortunately no consistent results obtained so far.

6.4 Clinical Manifestation and Diagnosis

6.4.1 What Are the Clinical Manifestations of KD

Since 1953, Yu Weihan (Fig. 6.6) and his team had detected more than 415 thousand cases and treated more than 3100 cases of KD patients in Heilongjiang, Jilin, Liaoning, Inner Mongolia, Hebei, Shandong and other provinces. Base on the above medical treatment experiences, corresponding follow-up observations, discussion with rural or country doctor, Yu Weihan comprehensively analyzed the clinical manifestations of KD and published a paper named of "The Concept of Keshan disease" in 1973.

According to the phase of onset and cardiac function, KD is divided into four types including acute type, sub-acute type, chronic type and latent type(Fig. 6.7). The chronic type, according to different states of cardiac function, is subdivided into chronic II, chronic III and chronic IV.

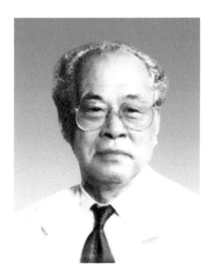

Fig. 6.6　Professor Weihan Yu, M. D. (1922-2010)

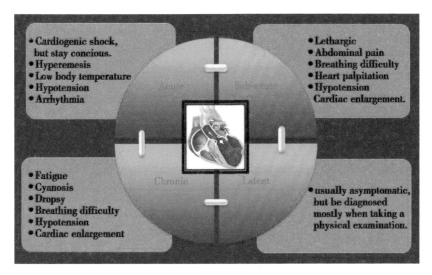

Fig. 6.7   Clinical classification for Keshan disease and major manifestations of each type.

Acute type is the main type of KD occurring in the northern China, more common in adults, fast onset and worsening rapidly. The major clinical manifestation is acute circulatory failure. Sub-acute type is more common in children living in the southwest of China and Shandong Province. The disease progression is slightly slow than acute type, but the major clinical manifestation also is acute heart failure.

Chronic type has occurred in all disease areas across the country involving both children and adults, which has become a major type of KD, clinically with chronic congestive heart failure as the main manifestation.

6. 4. 1. 1   Acute KD

Symptoms. Many patients feel general malaise, such as fatigue, limb weakness, dizziness, and heart discomfort prior to the onset of illness. Children often show lack of energy, irritability, crying, paroxysmal abdominal pain and polydipsia, etc. At the onset of KD the clinical manifestations are acute circulatory failure (cardiogenic shock), including nausea, vomiting, cough, asthma and thirst. Vomiting was projectile, frequent and intense, with spitting food scraps and acidic liquid firstly, and then yellow bile. Dyspnea can occur suddenly in some patients who cough up pink frothy sputum and feel anxious and fear. Other patients burst suddenly with syncope, seizures, cyanosis, cold limbs, and so on. Patients are generally alert. All acute-type KD patients will turn into chronic type if they can not be cured within three months.

Signs. The visible signs are acute circulatory failure, such as gray complexion, pale and slightly cyanotic lips, luster loss of skin, clammy body, cold extremities and low body temperature, pulselessness and even impalpable pulse, and rapid shallow breathing. In addition, blood pressure significantly reduces or even is difficult to be detected, and pulse pressure decreases. Apex beat is extremely weak or can not be touched. The heart border expands mildly toward left. Heart rate increases to above 100 beats per minute. The fastest one can be up to 200 times per minute. The diastolic gallop can be heard. The heart rate will decrease to under 50 in bradycardia and atrioventricular block. The lowest one is only a dozen times per minute, or even several times. Heart rhythm is often irregular, and typically changeable and varied, and even changes suddenly. There are serious lesions in the myocardium, so its contraction is weak, and first heart sound attenuates and is weak and deep, or even inaudible, especially in precordial region. The blowing systolic murmur below grade Ⅲ can be heard in the precordial region or apex of some patients' heart, and it is coarse, transient, and hard to be transmitted. In most patients, rhonchi and crackles can be heard in lung. In patients with pulmonary edema, blistering sound can be heard everywhere in both lungs, and wheezing rale can also be heard. Although its onset is rapid in some cases, it doesn't have serious condition. Therefore, it is called mild acute type, and its symptoms are similar to those of severe acute type, but lighter than it. The drop of blood pressure is not obvious and there is no serious arrhythmia.

6.4.1.2　Sub-acute KD

Symptoms. Lots of manifestations can be seen in the early stage. Common symptoms include cough, shortness of breath, lack of energy, unwillingness to play, sleepiness or crying, loss of appetite, thirst, intermittent abdominal pain, nausea, vomiting, ventosity and diarrhea. Symptoms caused by gastrointestinal infections firstly appear in some children, and abdominal pain, bloating, diarrhea are more obvious, followed by cough and asthma. Older kids often feel dizziness, headache, heart discomfort, weakness, palpitations, and so on. Some patients have mild fever. Heart failure occurs about one week later, and their condition rapidly deteriorates. Some symptoms such as cough, palpitations, and breathing difficulty get worse, and edema appears on eyelids, face and/or lower limb. In some patients, cerebral embolism is the main chief complaint or appears in the progression of their condition. In addition to the above symptoms, they also have embolism change, such as mouth crooked eye oblique, limb activity limitation, and sensory dysfunction.

Signs. In the early stage of children suffering from KD, the main signs are apathy, listless, pale or greenish yellow, slightly dark, eyelid edema, shortness of breath, and so on. With the further deterioration of patient's condition to heart failure, facial features of acute and serious illness are seen on children's face, accompanying other signs such as pale gray, extreme irritability, restlessness, severe dyspnea, cyanosis, facial swelling, aches and cold sweat, cold limbs, low body temperature, weak and rapid pulse, more than 50 times breathing of per minute, low blood pressure, and pulse pressure reduction even close to zero. Heart border moderately or significantly expands to both sides. Heart sounds are weakened, especially the first heart sound. Heart rate accelerates up to 100-160 beats per minute. Heart beat sounds are like pendulum frequency or diastolic gallop. Arrhythmia is not common. Moist rales is heard at the areas of two lungs. It shows a moderate degree of liver enlargement. Palpation of liver is soft and patients feel tenderness. There are also other signs such as jugular vein engorgement, positive signs of liver jugular venous return, lower extremity and/or systemic mild edema.

6.4.1.3 Chronic KD

Symptoms. All patients have insidious onset, and some patients can not describe the exact time of onset, which is called natural chronic type. Most chronic KD are evolved from other types in the high incidence of KD. Patients often have symptoms including dizziness, fatigue, loss of appetite, precordial discomfort, sometimes accompanied by nausea and vomiting. Heart palpitations, cough, shortness of breath, breathing difficulty, decreased urine output, facial or leg edema gradually appear after exertion. Some patients with paroxysmal nocturnal dyspnea cannot lie down, and have body swelling, whose sputum mixes blood streak. Such patients often have intractable heart failure, and seriously enlarged heart, and often die in the short term.

Signs. Patients showed signs of chronic tolerance, varying degrees of cyanosis, dull red cheeks, lip cyanosis, slightly lower blood pressure, pulselessness or irregularity, jugular varicosity, and other signs of systemic circulation congestion in different degrees. Mild cases only have edema of lower limbs, which is intermittent, mild in the morning and severe at night. Severe cases have serious edema of whole body, and even may have pleural, abdominal and pericardial effusion. Apex beat is diffused, and heart border moderately or seriously expands to both sides. The first heart sound may weaken, and blowing systolic murmur can be heard at the apex and anterior region of heart, some of which are up to above grade III, then diastolic gallop can be heard. Rhythm of the heart are often irregular, and premature beats and atrial fibrillation are common. Liver becomes moderately or observably swelling, and have tenderness. There are also other signs such as jugular vein engorgement, positive signs of liver and jugular venous return. Few patients have splenomegaly. It will be called acute exacerbation of chronic KD if there is acute onset of symptoms and signs.

6.4.1.4　Latent KD

There is generally no subjective symptom in latent KD due to mild myocardial lesions, lesser extent, preferable compensation of cardiac functions. Most of them are more able to participate in common physical labor, only diagnosed in the census or patient examination characterized by enlarged heart or ECG abnormalities. Some patients are transformed from other types of KD after treatment. A few patients feel dizziness, palpitations, nausea, discomfort after exertion, which will disappear after the break. Physical examination shows apex beat weakened, and mild expansion of cardiac dullness border to lower left. Sometimes, apex beat attenuates and blowing systolic murmur below grade III can be heard at anterior region of the heart. The heart rhythm is irregular and premature beats are more common.

6.4.2　What are the Laboratory Test Results of KD

6.4.2.1　Electrocardiography

Acute KD: Prolonged QT interval, low voltage of QRS wave group, and heart-block commonly appear in the early stage of acute type. S-T segment elevation shows an unidirectional, or ECG changes are similar to myocardial infarction in severe patients.

QRS wave is QR or Qr. It may be accompanied by arrhythmias. The most common change is premature ventricular contraction and atrioventricular block.

Sub-acute KD: Nodal tachycardia is common in sub-acute KD. Sometimes, ECG examination shows low voltage of QRS wave group, ST-T changes, atrioventricular block, right bundle branch block, ventricular premature, and S-T segment elevation like a single curve and necrotic Q waves. In the early onset, various abnormal ECGs are characterized by variability and irregularity.

Chronic KD: Almost all chronic KD patients have abnormal ECG, which include a variety of ECG changes. Sometimes, several anomalies can often coexist in one patient. The most common ECG abnormalities are ventricular premature, ST-T changes and right bundle branch block. Atrial premature, atrioventricular block, atrial fibrillation, and left atrial hypertrophy are also common. The detection rates of ventricular premature and ST-T changes are 40%-63.2% and 61%-79% respectively by ECG examination. This type of patients may be associated with ventricular premature (frequent, polygenetic, bigeminal, and ventricular tachycardia), ST-T changes, atrial fibrillation and complete right bundle branch block, and they have poor prognosis and shorter survival, especially while several anomalies coexist. The detection rate of ventricular premature, frequent ventricular premature, pair ventricular premature, non-paroxysmal ventricular tachycardia and atrial premature is 96.5%, 75.4%, 77.2%, 59.6% and 84.3% respectively. The characteristic of ventricular premature variation is periodic in 24h and like biological clock phenomenon.

Latent KD: The main changes of ECG examination are ventricular premature, incomplete right bundle branch block and/or ST-T changes. But the detection rate is lower than other types.

6.4.2.2 Chest Radiograph

Chest radiograph has important judgment value in the KD diagnosis and estimation of clinical outcome. Its main findings of KD are cardiac enlargement, weakened pulse, pulmonary congestion or pulmonary edema (Fig. 6.8).

Heart Size: The enlargement of heart suffering from KD is myogenic cardiac dilation. The outer edge of heart expands to both sides. Cardiac transverse diameter moves down. Heart phrenic angle widens. The biventricular types are

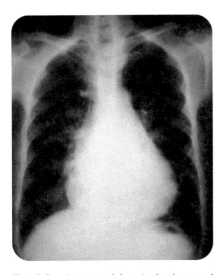

Fig. 6.8 Increased heart shadow and pulmonary congestion shown in chest radiograph of a patient with chronic Keshan disease.

more common heart shape and similar to flask or spherality. Sometimes, mitral valve type or aortic valve type may be visible. There are different degrees of enlargement in various chambers. The shape of pulmonary artery segment is straight or salient. The diameter of superior vena cava widens. Left ventricular enlargement is the most frequent in cardiomegaly. Meanwhile, the tip of the heart shifts to lower left. The secondary common part of heart enlargement is left atrium, while the right atrial enlargement is rare. Left ventricular enlargement commonly appears in mild cardiomegaly. However, all chambers of heart can be involved in obvious enlargement of heart.

Heart Beat: The heart beat is weak and irregular, which can be found by chest fluoroscopic examination. A few local pulses disappear and paradoxical pulsation appears. Heart kymogram photography can show that amplitude decreases or disappears.

Pulmonary Manifestations: Pulmonary congestion, pulmonary edema, lung field blur, and interstitial and alveolar edema are common representations in acute or sub-acute KD. In chronic cases, lung congestion frequently appears, while lung markings increase, thicken, extend, and blur.

6.4.2.3 Echoardiography

The internal diameter of left ventricle, left atrium, and right ventricular commonly increases, but it's rare in the right atrium. The detection rate of increasing diameter is the highest in left ventricle, followed by the left atrium and right ventricle.

The pulsating amplitude of aorta, ventricular septal and left ventricular posterior wall are reduced. M-type cardiac echoardiography shows decreasing motion amplitudes of anterior mitral valve, and widening left ventricular outflow tract,similar to a small prism.

The thickness of ventricular septum and left ventricular posterior wall may be normal or thinning. The latter is quite common in patients whose hearts are obviously dilated. The regional motion abnormality of ventricular wall can occur, especially at the apex of heart.

The heart function generally decreases. A peak is larger than E peak in mitral inflow. The ejection fraction (EF%) and myocardial fractional shortening (FS%) are smaller.

6.4.2.4　Blood and Urine Tests

Serum Myocardial Enzyme Changes: The activity of serum glutamic-oxaloacetic transaminase (SGOT), creatine phosphokinase (CPK) and its isoenzyme, lactate dehydrogenase (LDH) and its isoenzyme can increase in varying degrees in acute and sub-acute KD. They often begin to increase hours later of the onset, reach the peak from 1 to 3 days, and then gradually return to normal level after 1 to 2 weeks. They also increase in various degrees at acute exacerbation of chronic KD. The change of serous myocardial enzymes is an important value to diagnose KD and evaluate myocardial damage. For example, it indicates new myocardial damage that there is an increase of myocardial enzymes activity in convalescence sub-acute KD.

Other Blood Indice Examination: There isn't an obvious change of red blood cell counts and hemoglobin in all KD. The count of leukocytes and granulocyte increases in a part of acute and sub-acute patients. Chronic type patients often have varying degrees of anemia and their erythrocyte sedimentation rate increases. The analysis of serum protein shows low serum albumin and increased globulin in chronic KD.

Urinalysis: There is no obvious specific change in urinalysis in KD, and only chronic KD has proteinuria.

6.4.3　What Evidences are Required for KD Diagnosis

There isn't a specific diagnostic method for KD, which is diagnosed mainly after precluding other diseases. Based on the KD Diagnostic Criteria (GB17021-1997), KD can be diagnosed by meeting the following three criteria: (1) Having epidemiological characteristics of KD in specific areas, duration and population. The immigrant population can only suffer from KD by living in the same way of life as local farmers for three consecutive months in the disease area; (2) Having signs and symptoms of heart disease, cardiomegaly and/or ECG abnormalities, or symptoms and signs of heart failure, including heart palpitations, shortness of breath, gallop, hepatomegaly, and edema; (3) Exclusion of other cardiac diseases.

Precluding other diseases, KD can be diagnosed if there is one of the following characteristics:

1) Cardiomegaly by physical examination, chest radiograph and echocardiography
2) Acute or chronic cardiac dysfunction
3) Arrhythmia
   (a) Multiple ventricular premature, more than six times per minute, increasing after exercise
   (b) Atrial fibrillation
   (c) Paroxysmal supra-ventricular or ventricular tachycardia
4) Gallop
5) Embolism of brain or other organs
6) ECG abnormality
   (a) Atrioventricular heart-block
   (b) Bundle branch block,apart from incomplete right bundle branch block
   (c) ST-T changes
   (d) Q-T interval prolongation
   (e) Multiple or polygenic premature ventricular contractions
   (f) Paroxysmal supra-ventricular or ventricular tachycardia
   (g) Atrial fibrillation or atrial flutter
   (h) P-wave abnormalities, and left, right, or both atrial enlargement
7) Chest Radiograph finding: cardiomegaly
8) Echocardiography, including Doppler echocardiography
   (a) Increasing diameter of left atrium and left ventricle
   (b) Ejection fraction (EF%) down to 40% or less
   (c) Regional wall motion abnormality
   (d) A peakbeing greater than E peak in mitral valve flow spectrum
9) Myocardial enzyme changes, mainly used to diagnose acute or sub-acute type patient

（a） GOT activity increase, GOT/GPT> 1

（b） LDH and LDH1 increase

（c） CK and its isoenzyme activity increase

6. 4. 4　How to Identify KD among Similar Cardiomyopathies

KD is easily confused with a variety of diseases and can be identified through careful medical history inquiry, physical examination and necessary laboratory tests. Acute KD needs to be differentiated from acute myocarditis, acute myocardial infarction, and acute gastritis. It is necessary to differentiate sub-acute KD from bronchial pneumonia, acute or chronic glomerulonephritis, or chronic kidney disease. Dilated cardiomyopathy（DCM）, ischemic and peripartum cardiomyopathy should be differentiated from Chronic type. Otherwise, we must differentiate latent type from focal myocarditis, hypertrophic non-infarct cardiomyopathy and nonspecific ECG changes.

6. 4. 4. 1　Identification of Acute KD

Acute Myocarditis: Signs of acute myocarditis are manifested as palpitations, chest pain, dyspnea and edema. We found accelerated heart rate, arrhythmia, edema by physical examination. Heart size is normal or mild to moderate increase by chest radiograph. ECG examination shows ST-T changes, premature beat, and conduction block. All these are similar to KD. Acute myocarditis is caused by viral infection. The patients often feel fatigue, nausea, and vomiting like influenza during 1 to 2 weeks prior to the onset. The number of leukocytes reduces and the Lymphocyte fraction increases. The antibody titers are more than four times higher than that before onset in double serum tests. Virus, virus gene or viral protein antigen can be detected from endocardial, myocardial, and pericardial puncture fluid during the acute phase. The increase of enzyme activity isn't significant as compared to KD. Therefore, identification of two diseases can be based on these characteristics.

　　Acute Myocardial Infarction: The onset of acute myocardial infarction is abrupt accompanied by cardiogenic shock, severe heart failure and arrhythmias and ST-T changes of ECG, especially similar unindirectional curve to KD. However, acute myocardial infarction patients are relatively older. They often have hypertension, hyperlipidemia, obesity history, and so on, and often feel angina or precordial discomfort. There is an obviously evolutionary process from damage, necrosis to ischemia on ECG. It is more common among male patients.

Acute Gastritis: Patients of acute gastritis often feel abdominal discomfort, nausea, vomiting, fatigue, cold limbs, and sometimes spit bile, etc. These signs are similar to KD. However, acute gastritis patients have the history of engorgement or eating contaminated food, accompanied by abdominal pain, diarrhea, without cardiac signs. There aren't cardiac abnormalities by Chest Radiograph and ECG. According these differences acute gastritis can be distinguished.

6. 4. 4. 2　Identification of Sub-acute KD

Nephritis Pyelonephritis: Nephritis pyelonephritis in children is apt to be confused with sub-acute KD due to similar swelling, especially facial swelling accompanied by heart failure. We can differentiate it from sub-acute KD based on high blood pressure, protein in urine, hematuria or urine casts.

Bronchial Pneumonia: Children with bronchial pneumonia complicated by heart failure, who have signs of dyspnea, irritability, rapid heart rate, hepatomegaly or edema, are often confused with sub-acute KD, especially pediatric patients accompanied by pulmonary infection. It is easy to identify them by the presence of fever, obvious pulmonary rhonchi or crackles, increase of total white blood cells, particularly neutrophils, mostly normal size of heart and sinus tachycardia.

In addition, sub-acuteKD also needs to be discriminated from myocarditis, referring to differential diagnosis of acute KD.

6. 4. 4. 3　Identification of Chronic KD

Dilated Cardiomyopathy (**DCM**): DCM patients have insidious onset, cardiomegaly, heart failure, arrhythmias, jugular varicosity, hepatomegaly, lower extremity or whole body edema. All these clinical manifestations are extremely similar to KD. Thus, a differentiation of them is very difficult. In chronic KD patients, premature ventricular contractions and complete right bundle branch block are more common, while atrial fibrillation and left ventricular hypertrophy are more common in DCM. As patients from KD endemic and/or Kashin-Beck disease area, especially those with acute or sub-acute type history can make a diagnosis of KD. Natural chronic type is mainly based on disease characteristics distinction.

Ischemic Cardiomyopathy: Patients of ischemic cardiomyopathy have several similar clinical manifestations to KD, such as cardiomegaly, heart failure, arrhythmia, hepatomegaly, lower extremity or whole body edema. It can be differentiated from KD based on the history of coronary heart disease, the older age of incidence, and abnormalities of lipid and lipoprotein, including increased cholesterol, triglycerides and low density lipoprotein, reduced high-density lipoprotein, and vascular sclerosis or valvular calcification by chest radiograph and echoardiography, etc.

Others: Women in reproductive ages are the main KD population and should be differentiated from peripartum cardiomyopathy. It can be done based on its relationship with childbirth. In addition, Chronic KD can also be discriminated from mitral inadequacy of rheumatic heart disease based on its history, cardiac souffle, and valve changes in ultrasonic examination, especially increased murmur after heart failure being controlled.

6.4.4.4　Identification of Latent KD

Focal Myocarditis: There is ventricular premature in ECG of focal myocarditis due to inflammatory reaction, scarring and fibrosis. These are also the common manifestations of latent KD. The main difference between them is that focal myocarditis has the characteristics of viral infection, referencing to acute KD.

Hypertrophic Non-Obstructive Cardiomyopathy: Like latent KD, there are thickening of ventricular septum and left ventricular wall in hypertrophic non-obstructive cardiomyopathy. However, these patients often feel precordial pain and discomfort, having coarse systolic bruit, significant thickening of ventricular septum and left ventricular wall, and characteristics of left ventricular hypertrophy or abnormal Q-wave in ECG. All these can be helpful to differentiate them.

Nonspecific ECG Changes: Most patients of latent type KD often haven't had any subjective symptom, with only several abnormalities of ECG, such as I° atrial ventricular block, frequent ventricular premature, and ST-T changes in physical examination. These changes are not unique to KD. Thus, other causes should be ruled out.

I° atrial ventricular block may be found in the healthy young population. Its detection rate is from 0.65% to 1.1%, approximately 1.3% in the age above 50 years. It is mainly caused by the increase of the vagus nerve tension, sometimes, which can also lead to secondary degree I type A-V block. Both can be dispelled after serving atropine or exercise. Frequent ventricular premature and ST-T changes can be found in a variety of structural heart disease, electrolyte imbalance, drug toxicity, etc. These confounding factors can be differentiated respectively by having features of primary heart disease, abnormal blood parameters, and taking or exposed to relative medication. Frequent ventricular premature may also be functional and can disappear after activity.

6.5 Cardiac Histopathology

The pathological change of KD mainly involves the myocardium, showing severe degeneration, necrosis, fibrous scar recovery, etc. (Fig. 6.9). Skeletal muscle can also be involved, but the extent of lesion is light. Other organs of the body also have different degrees of pathological changes, which are mainly secondary to acute and chronic heart dysfunction.

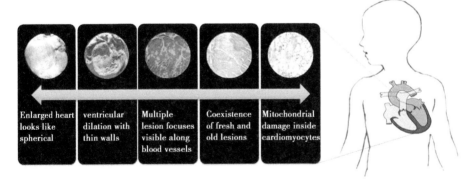

| Enlarged heart looks like spherical | ventricular dilation with thin walls | Multiple lesion focuses visible along blood vessels | Coexistence of fresh and old lesions | Mitochondrial damage inside cardiomyocytes |

Fig. 6.9　Abnormal cardiac morphology in KD patients.

6.5.1　What are Cardiac Images under Macroscopic Observation

6.5.1.1　Heart Size

Cardiac dilatation. The heart has a different degree of dilatation in all KD patients, except a very small number of acute patients with a short course or latent KD patients without cardiac dysfunction. The largest is up to 2 to 3 times as normal heart, especially in chronic KD. The cardiac dilatation of children with chronic KD is more significant, even causes the precordial uplift or thoracic deformation in more serious patients（Fig. 6.10）.

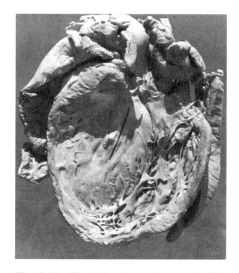

Fig. 6.10 Typical enlarged heart of a 59-year-old man died of chronic Keshan disease.

The dilatation of the heart is mainly caused by myocardial metamorphism, scarring, muscle fiber stretching and leng-th-ening（myogenic dilatation）secondary to repeated myocardial deterioration. In a certain extent, the cardiac hypertrophy is covered by the remarkable dilatation of the cardiac cavity, which is not obvious. The longitudinal and transverse diameters of heart are increased in KD patients, so the heart loses its original oblate tapered shape and change to spherical or almond shape.

The degree of KD heart weight gain is usually less than its dilation. In the acute KD with serious necrosis, heart weight is about 250-350 grams. In chronic KD with long course, there is a widespread myocardial fibrous scar, cardiac hypertrophy, and significant dilatation of heart cavity, and the heart weight can exceed 500 grams or more. Children with chronic type can reach 2-3 times as the heart weight of the same age children.

6.5.1.2 Ventricular Wall

The ventricle wall of KD heart usually dose not show incrassation, or even attenuation. A great number of lesions with clear edges are visible in sections of the ventricular wall. Three types of myocardial lesion are observed with naked eyes. First, myocardial section has a greyish yellow color, lacking luster, and not being sunken, whose texture is soft and flabby, flaky or plaque. The chief manifestation of pathological change is necrosis. While left ventricle is sectioned longitudinally, subendocardial lesions are observed and often distributed in the circumferential wall of the heart. Sometimes, the necrosis area is surrounded by hyperaemia and hemorrhage, with clear boundaries, similar to the infarct necrosis. Second, the myocardial section is dark gray, and slightly concave, with a slight transparency. The boundary of this kind of lesion is very clear, patchy or of short cords, and its fibrous scar lesions are fresh, from absorbed lesions to early recovery stage. Third, the myocardial section is going grey, and depression. Its quality is hard, and it is a massive or dendritic irregular scar, which belongs to the old scar. The above pathological changes can be present in the same case. The left ventricular and ventricular septum are more serious than the right ventricle, and the inner layer of the myocardium, papillary muscle and the middle layer are more serious than outer layer.

6.5.1.3 Endocardium

Plaque thickening can be seen in endocardium, and mural thrombus is always observed. There is no obvious change observed by naked eye in the endocardium of acute and sub-acute KD. Mild diffuse incrassation and turning white of left ventricle endocardium can be observed in KD patients with longer duration and significant cardiac dilatation. In the patients with chronic type, the white verrucous thickening is easily seen in the left ventricular intima, which is caused by the organization of mural thrombus, covering its surface. The mural thrombus is always observed in various types of cases, whose predilection sites are left ventricle, left and right atrial appendage.

Each valve is usually normal. In chronic type with obvious heart dilation, the mitral valve is relatively insufficient. Nonspecific thickening and rolling up at the free edge of the mitral valve with smooth surface could be visualized, caused by blood adverse current.

6.5.1.4 Epicardium

Focal or diffuse pericardial adhesions of epicardium are observed in some cases, with a narrow band of necrosis area close to the outer membrane. A small amount of epicardial fibrin exudes at epicardium, proliferating of granulation tissue.

6.5.2 What are Cardiac Images under Microscopic Observation

6.5.2.1 Myocardial Parenchymal Degeneration

Granular Degeneration: The fibril of cardiac muscle is swollen, with unclear transverse striation. The myofibril is interrupted, with fine particle spreading.

Regularly arranged myofibril contraction bands appear in the muscle fibers of severe lesions, and its width varies. Myofibril is broken and characterized by coarse granular structure, developing to myocardial coagulation necrosis.

Vesicular Degeneration: The fibril of cardiac muscle is slightly swollen, and small cavities with blurred boundary are visible in endochylema stained slightly. Myofibrillar is vaguely discernible. The myofibril is sparse. Vacuoles fuse each other. Nucleus is swelled. The nucleolus is obviously seen. The chromatin is margination. It ends with myofibrillar lysis and necrosis after the lesion is gradually increased.

Fatty Degeneration: The lipid droplets are small and neatly arranged when lesion is mild. It becomes large with lesion aggravation. The stripes of myofibrils are not clear. The lipid droplets coarse fibrils and stripes are unclear. Lipid droplets are distributed in a range of foci, and are parallel to the severity of myocardial injury. In the semi thin sections, visible osmic acid staining of lipid droplets appears between the myofibrils. The size of lipid droplets ranges from 0.5 to 4μm in diameter, which are found in acute cases.

6.5.2.2 Myocardial Necrosis

Myocardial necrosis is divided into two basic types: coagulation and liquefaction. The common points between the two types include myocardial fiber necrosis, residual mesenchyme and inflammation caused by absorptive and reparative response.

Coagulative Myocytolysis: Coagulative myocytolysis refers to a series of changes occurring in myocardial cells, including myofibril disintegration and condensation, myocardial fiber swelling, myofibril coagulation, and showing homogeneous and structureless nodular mass or shape of cross strip. Damaged myocardium with irregular margin is easier to be enzymatic hydrolyzed and liquefied, which has a low homogeneous degree, and poor refraction, with a high content of cell infiltration. Necrosis material is consumed and absorbed through enzymatic hydrolyzed by macrophage left behind spongy empty frame after necrosis.

Colliquative Myocytolysis: Colliquative myocytolysis means that the myocardial fibers are filled with more liquid. There are numerous vacuoles in the cytoplasm, and the myofibers are loose and scattered, stained slightly, gradually disappearing, replaced by huge vacuole, and showing peripheral interstitial bracket. At this point the nucleus of cardiac myocyte is swelling and has vacuolization. Myofibrils, mitochondria and other organelles are widely dissolved, and eventually the whole muscle fiber develops into a cavity and the lesions become mesh like empty frame. In this type of necrosis, inflammatory reaction is usually not obvious, and the fibroblast is also less at a later stage, replaced with the formation of scar mainly through the collagenzation of reticular fibers.

The Distribution of Myocardial Necrosis: The distribution of myocardial necrosis shows multiple focal features, separated by normal myocardial tissue. The shape of myocardial necrosis lesion may be punctate, miliary, and patchy after fusion or infarct like necrosis. The basic form of myocardial necrosis is multiple miliary. The most obvious difference with other myocardium necrosis is a fairly large number of similarly sized lesion, dispersed on the whole layers. The larger necrotic lesions often tend to be centrifugal. There are many inflammatory cells and residual myocardial cells in the peripheral part of the lesions. Slightly inside are varying degrees of myocardial vesicular degeneration, muscle dissolution and hollow frame after necrosis. The central focus of lesion is the fibrous connective tissue. The infarct like necrosis is composed of uniform large empty frame after necrosis, or integrated by many smaller patches of necrosis. The narrow and incomplete myocardial strip is sometimes shown near endocardium.

Myocardial damage occurs in groups, and can coexists with old and new lesions (Fig. 6.11). The coexistence of new and old lesions is sequentially from left ventricular to the right chamber, and from the inner layer to the outer. In the same position, old lesions commonly exist in the center, and fresh necrosis are surrounding. The coexistence of the new and old lesion is common in adults of KD living in northern area. However, the lesion is mainly consistent in sub-acute KD occurring in southern children.

The distribution of necrosis focus is

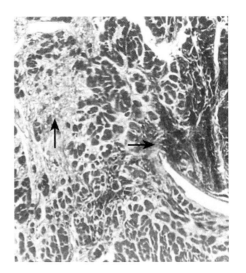

Fig. 6.11   Concurrent old and fresh necrosis focuses shown within myocardium of Keshan disease.

closely related to the course of myocardial coronary artery, and there are two common types of peri-vascular necrosis (Fig. 6.12). One type of peri-vascular necrosis is relevant to branching vessel, and miliary necrosis focus is located in the innervate regions of coronary artery. This kind of lesions shows cluster distribution, clear frontier, similar size, spherical shape, and is scattered in all layer of the muscle wall. It seems peculiarly like a bunch of grapes and is the most common lesions. Another type of peri-vascular necrosis is interr-elated to

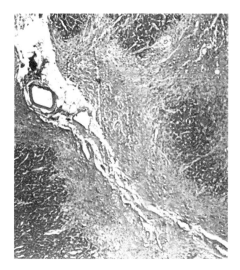

Fig. 6.12　Perivascular myocardial lesions seen in Keshan diseased heart.

straight type vessel and is mainly around straight or branched stems of the main coronary artery. The width of lesion varies from one or two layers of myocardial fibers (narrow sleeves) to multi-layered muscle bundles. It can also be composed of several incomplete miliary focal foci scattered on both sides of the vessel. Such lesion can occur under the epicardium or in myocardium around a certain segment of blood vessel lying in middle heart wall, and may also be associated with an entire straight trunk forming a wide sleeve peri-vascular lesion. There are two main forms of peri-vascular morphology located in the left ventricular papillary muscle necrosis foci. In the dendritic papillary muscles, the myocardial necrotic lesions across the papillary muscle are distributed along the vessel, alternately distributed with healthy myocardium. In the finger papillary muscles, myocardial necrotic lesions form small and irregular tigroid necrosis in which transverse arteries are visible. For the site of occurrence, the lesion is located around the end of arterial through the microcirculation bed. There is a low density of blood vessel in this area.

6.5.2.3　Inflammatory Reaction

With the progress of myocardial necrosis, there are varying degrees of interstitial inflammatory reactions due to necrosis, which is not obvious in the early stage. In severe necrosis, a certain number of lymphocytes can be detected. When the necrosis is acute and severe, there are more neutrophils, lymphocytes and monocytes appearing around necrotic myocardial fibers. At the same time, inflammation is also comparatively obvious in interstitial and perivascular tissue. However, there are only a small number of inflammatory cells infiltrated in myocardium away from the necrotic area. The main characteristics of KD is the progress of myocardial degeneration, necrosis and rehabilitation, while the inflammation belongs to the absorption reaction of phagocytosis.

The inflammatory reaction at the endocardium and epicardium of KD is mild, and limited, with lymph and mononuclear cell mainly infiltrating in small focus. The inflammation is only comparatively obvious when myocardial necrosis appears. There are more inflammatory cells in endocardium adjacent to organized lateral thrombus.

6.5.2.4　Rehabilitation and Regeneration

In KD, rehabilitation of myocardial necrosis foci is mainly replaced with scar tissue formatted by hyperplastic reticular fiber, which usually does not form extensive interstitial fibrosis. Many healthy myocardiums are extant among focal scars. Sometimes, there is a net formed by finespun collagenous fiber bundle trapping cardiac muscle fibers.

The regenerated cardiomyocytes often appear in the lesion during reparative process from the late stage of necrosis to the early stage of scarring. The cells are stained with alkaline. Their strips are blurry and unclear. Their nuclei are generally increasing. Binucleate cells and polykaryocyte are common. There are often various degrees of cardiomyocytes hypertrophy around scars in the case which scars are mainly in the late stage.

6.5.2.5　Myocardial Conduction System Changes

KD lesions often involve the interventricular septum, especially the cardiac muscle of endocardium. The conduction system may be also involved. Denaturation, necrosis and fibrosis are the main characteristics of conduction system lesions. It's most severe on the both branches of bundle. The right bundle branches are often interrupted. His Bundle and atrioventricular node are damaged slightly. There is generally no change in sinoatrial node.

6.5.3   What are the Pathological Changes of Other Tissues and Organs

6.5.3.1   Striated Muscle

In some cases of Keshan disease, there are also similar lesions to myocardium in striated muscle. But the degree of lesion is mild and there is no obvious change in gross appearance. Under the microscope, we can observe denaturation, necrosis, and then inflammatory cells infiltrating, phagorytosis and absorption, rehabilitation and regeneration of muscle fibers in single or small muscle group, in which there is tiny scar. The lesions mainly involve the diaphragm, intercostal muscle, gastrocnemius muscle and lingualis.

6.5.3.2   Lung

There are different degrees of acute or chronic pulmonary congestion in patientswith KD. Some patients are accompanied with edema, transudative hemorrhage, and a few cases with fresh or obsolete infarction. Sub-acute KD is often complicated by interstitial pneumonia. Its autopsy detection rate was from 50% to 90%.

6.5.3.3   Liver

There are nearly half of chronic cases with different degrees of fibrosis after hepatic congestion, of which a few cases have developed to congestive cirrhosis. The acute type of persistent cardiac shock and hypotension often cause the central infarct like necrosis of hepatic lobule. The extent of the lesion was positively correlated with the severity and duration of shock.

Pathological changes of other organs are secondary to heart failure and mural thrombus.

6.5.4   What is the Relationship between Clinic and Pathology?

At present, the popular clinical type of KD is mainly based on the cardiac function in patients. However, there are differences in the main characteristics of lesions and the severity of the disease. The general characteristics of the clinical types are listed as follows.

6.5.4.1   Acute Type

The main characteristics of myocardial lesions are degeneration and necrosis, commonly taking place under endocardium. It is often shown as yellow patches lesionsunder gross observation. The cardiac dilatation and weight gain is generally mild and the shape of heart can be maintained. Myocardial scar is few and small. Acute congestion and edema of organs are the secondary changes to acute shock.

6.5.4.2 Sub-acute Type

The myocardial pathological changes of sub-acute Keshan disease are generally residual framework after necrosis and unconsolidated scar in the early stage. The lesion is often more extensive and with the representative perivascular phenomenon. Under gross observation, there are sharp-edged, translucent and small lesions in myocardium. They form uneven patches in the left ventricular papillary muscle. The increase of cardiac diameter and weight is significantly more obvious than that in acute type. Consequent changes of congestive heart failure are found in all organs.

6.5.4.3 Chronic Type

In chronic KD, cardiac lesions are mainly dated scars. The weight of heart is significantly increased. The myocardial fibers have undergone hypertrophy, especially around scars. The ventricular dilatation is significant, and papillary muscle and trabeculum are flat. There are chronic congestions in various organs.

6.5.4.4 Latent Type

There aren't obvious signs or symptoms in latent KD due to an initial stage of the lesion. Another possibility is the myocardial damage has been rehabilitated because of occult onset. It is occasionally found in the autopsy of a few cases that there are different degrees of cardiac pathological changes. The range of lesion is small, and the increase of diameter and weight of heart is not obvious.

6.6 Therapies

A general clinical treatment principle for KD is to improve myocardial metabolism, to control heart failure, to correct arrhythmia, to recover cardiac function, and to keep long-term treatment during recovery, despite significant differences of its four types in pathological changes and clinical manifestations. The outbreak patterns of KD have been greatly changed, from largely acute and sub-acute type during past years to be current chronic and latent type after 1980.

In addition, remarkable progress has been made in pharmacotherapy for patients with chronic KD due to the worldwide revolutionary understanding of chronic heart failure.

6.6.1 Treatment of Patients with Acute KD

A basic principle including early detection, diagnosis and treatment plus on-site rescue is recommended for patients with acute KD, who usually should stay in bed, keeping still and inhaling oxygen. Subhibernation therapy is useful for dysphoria patients in critical conditions, helping to reduce the basal metabolic rate, and to promote cardiac function recovery. Fortunately, mega-dose intravenous vitamin C therapy created by Dr. Shichen Wang (Fig. 6. 13) at then Xi'an Medical College as first-line treatment choice has a powerful effect on correcting myocardial ischemia and hypoxia, relieving the cardiac shock. After having the emergency condition to be controlled, clinical physician should provide life guidance for the patients, requiring a good rest, and having a checkup every three months to avoid turning into chronic type.

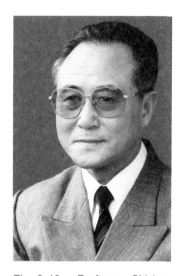

Fig. 6.13   Professor Shichen Wang, M.D. (1926-2003)

A practical protocol for mega-dose intravenous vitamin C therapy is: 5 to 10 grams of 10-12.5% vitamin C injection alone or together with 20 ml of 25-50% glucose solution are needed to be injected straight into a patient's vein. After 2 to 4 hours, the same thing can be repeatedly undertaken for once or twice depending on his or her condition. On day 1 of the treatment, a total administration dose of vitamin C can reach as much as 30g. Following mitigation of cardiogenic shock, a daily injection of 5 grams of vitamin C is necessary for 3-5 consecutive days. Pediatric dosage of vitamin C is 3 to 5 grams every day.

If the shock occurs again, a repeated application of mega-dose intravenous vitamin C therapy will be encouraged, which can restore approximately 50 to 60% of low blood pressure and arrhythmia in critical conditions. For severe heart failures, instant digitalis preparations such as Cedilanid at a dosage of 0.2mg/time or 0.125 mg/time of Strophanthus are administrated by vein.

6. 6. 2　Treatment of Patients with Sub-acute and Chronic KD

Treatment for early onset of a sub-acute patient refers to that for acute cases, but the therapy should be immediately turned to that for chronic type once the condition becomes chronic heart failure. General treatment principle is to remove major precipitating factors, to control heart failure, to correct arrhythmia, and to improve myocardial metabolism. In clinical practice, medications such as diuretics, positive inotropic drugs, angiotensin converting enzyme inhibitors (ACEI) and angiotensin II receptor antagonist (ARB), beta blockers, and anti-arrhythmic drugs are usually taken. For patients with cardiac function grade NYHA III and grade NYHA IV, they should be hospitalized for treatment. For patients with cardiac function grade NYHA II as well as those during recovery, treatment programs include domestic sickbed and regular follow-up.

A combined pharmacotherapy uses ACEI at first, and then beta blockers that can be added at the dose escalation phase of ACEI or depends on clinical conditions. For patients with cardiac function grade NYHA II, the principal consideration is to use ACEI and beta blockers in combination. While for patients with cardiac function grade NYHA III, they can be used together with diuretics and/or positive inotropic drugs at the same time. But for patients with cardiac function grade NYHA IV, they should be used after cardiac function improvement as a result of the application of diuretics and positive inotropic drugs. Much detailed approaches are described as below.

(1) To avoid or control precipitating factors listed as follows: overloading work, high stress, dietary consumption of high sodium salt, getting pregnant under ill condition, upper respiratory tract infection or pulmonary infection in cold weather, long-term unbalanced diet, and habitual overeating.

(2) Usage of diuretics: This kind of medicines can usually be used together with other drugs, not as a single choice for treatment. Administration of diuretics should start from a lower dose, for example Hydrochlorothiazide at 25mg per day and Furosemide at 20mg per day, gradually boosting dose until the appearance of

urine output increment. Body weight change is a reliable indicator monitoring the effect of a diuretic and its dose adjustment, with weight loss of 0.5 to 1.0kg every day reaching a stable condition for the treated patient. Subsequently, the minimum dose of a diuretic is needed to maintain a long-term treatment effect. Be careful of induced adverse effects, for instance, electrolyte imbalance, which needs timely supplement of potassium and sodium.

（3） Usage of angiotensin converting enzyme inhibitors （ACEI）: In clinical practice, some drugs such as Captopril, Enalapril, and Benazepril are commonly used for chronic heart failure. As top priority drugs for chronic cardiac insufficiency of KD, ACEI's administration in combination with diuretics, digitalis and beta blockers can provide synergetic effect, suitable for long-term treatment of the patients with cardiac function grade NYHA II, III, IV, as well as asymptomatic left ventricular systolic dysfunction. Beginning with a small dose of ACEI, its dose is escalated for 5 to 7 days up to the target dose, which will be taken for a long term. The therapeutic effect would work in a couple of months or longer time. It is ok for the transient intolerance to ACEI among some of the patients in the process of increasing doses, as long as systolic blood pressure value of patients is not less than 90 mmHg.

（4） Usage of beta blockers: Beta blocker therapy represents a major advance in the treatment of heart failure patients. This sort of drugs can be categorized by non-selective agents, selective agents and agents with vasodilatory effect. The mechanisms include up-regulation of beta receptor, reversing remodeling, improving contractile and diastolic function, antiarrhythmia and anti-ischemia. Evidences from randomized controlled clinical trials have supported its use in the treatment of patients with heart failure to decrease mortality and improve life quality. Guidelines with various versions recommend that beta blockers are indicated for patients with symptomatic or asymptomatic heart failure and ejection fraction lower than 40% .It should be noticed for the rational use of beta blockers such as timing, dosage, duration and contraindications.

Long-term use of beta blockers for patients with KD can lower fatality rate and prolongs survival period as conventional drugs for clinical application, largely specific beta 1 and concurrent receptor blockers are taken, for example, Metoprolol, Bisoprolol and Carvedilol. The use of beta blockers should be medically individualized because of the notable difference of patients' reaction to it. Beta blockers are inapplicable to the spasm of coronary vein, bradycardia (heart rate less than 60 times/min), high-degree atrioventricular block, hypotension, bronchospasm, obstructive lung disease, and intermittent claudication.

(5) Clinical application of positive inotropic drugs: Some frequently used digitalis preparation like Digoxin, Lanatoside, and Strophanthus K are capable of boosting the tolerance of patients to exercise, being good for moderate to severe heart failure (cardiac function grade NYHA III and IV) with quick sinus rhythm or rapid supraventricular arrhythmia in ECG, and the therapeutic effect may be even better if digitalis is combined with diuretic, ACEI, ARB, and beta-blockers. For mild heart failure (cardiac function grade NYHA II), digitalis drugs can be taken in the case of persistent symptoms despite having administered diuretics and ACEI. However, digitalis drugs are not recommended for systolic heart failure in asymptomatic individuals, and absolutely forbidden for those with conduction block. On the other hand, attention should be paid to excess or poisoning issue in the clinical use of digitalis due to its rather narrow range of effective amount and toxic dose, as well as imparity of individual sensitivity to it, particularly in children.

Besides, there are non-digitalis medicines classified into two families, i. e., β adrenergic receptor agonists and phosphodiesterase inhibitors (PDEI). Dobutamine and Dopamine, as primary drugs in receptor agonists family, can be used in mixture, beginning with small doses, performing significant therapeutic effect on low cardiac output, high left ventricular filling pressure, and hypotension. PDEI are just taken as optional drugs for a short-term use after treatment failure of combined application of diuretic, digoxin and vasodilator, seeking for the last treatment chance.

(6) Clinical application of anti-arrhythmic drugs: The arrhythmia induced by heart failure often fades out after cardiac function improvement. If arrhythmia is caused by primary myocardial injury, cardioversion would be needed by administrating Amiodarone, one of the best anti-arrhythmic drugs. Pacemaker installation may be the only effective way for curing the patients with persistent tardy arrhythmia, whose heart rate is lower than 40 times every minute. For patients with refractory heart failure after failed treatment by internal medicine, a surgery of heart transplantation will be the last choice.

6. 6. 3 Treatment of Patients with Latent KD

Usually no special treatment is required for latent patients because of better cardiac compensatory function, but some cares are needed for proper arrangement of daily life, work and rest, getting rid of infection factors. However, those patients who have slight enlargement of heart, ST-T changes or ventricular premature beat in their ECGs should get a prolonged clinical management. Especially the patients with serious myocardial injury, whose latent type is a treatment outcome of acute type, sub-acute type or chronic type, need enough time to recover. Long-term use of ACEI (Angiotensin Converting Enzyme Inhibitors), beta blockers, Vitamin C, and other drugs are helpful for the latent patients who constantly suffer from myocardial damage. To keep track of the prognosis, regular follow-up is a necessary step.

6. 6. 4 Precaution of Sudden Death Induced by KD

Sudden death is the second leading cause for all death cases of KD, and the crucial approach for its precaution is to control conduction block factors, which may induce ventricular arrhythmias and slow heart beat. Specifically, some steps include: (a) to keep away induced arrhythmia by reducing ventricular wall stress to prevent heart failure; (b) to correct neuroendocrine dysfunction by administration of ACEI and beta blockers; (c) to avoid drug factors such as the side effects of digitalis and diuretics, especially keep from the addiction of digitalis preparations.

6. 6. 5 Assessment of Therapeutic Effect

It's important, under normal circumstances, to track the outcomes of patients who have received certain treatment. To achieve this goal, we ought to carry out a comparative analysis on changes of clinical manifestations from patients with KD before and after the administration of a preventive measure or a drug, according to the indicators in the *Criteria for Evaluating Therapeutic Effect of KD* (*WS/T 209-2001*).

6. 7 Prevention Measures

A variety of measures employed for KD prevention not only aim at preventing it from occurring, but also effectively block or delay the pathogenic process for reducing tissue or organ injury. Here we adopt the three-grade prevention methodology: the primary prevention is targeting causal factors of KD; the secondary prevention mainly includes early detection, diagnosis and treatment of KD, improving its cure rate and reducing fatality rate; the tertiary prevention refers to symptomatic treatment and rehabilitation for chronic patients with bad prognosis of KD.

Practically, as low living level for most patient families, the best way of tertiary prevention of KD is home sickbed model, which has yet been widely taken in China. We have obtained satisfactory results from a Self-Management Program in 2005 for patients with chronic KD involving Shandong and Inner Mongolia. In addition, the scope of this program was expanded to eight provinces in the following year, and a preliminary conclusion was that those patients, who were compliant to the medical requests, usually received better therapeutic effects. Proper treatment of chronic KD can improve cardiac function, effectively inhibits progression of the disease and significantly reduces fatality rate. This program plays an important role in mitigating community pressure, maintaining social stability, promoting local economic development, and getting rid of family poverty. In view of the curability and actual therapeutic effect of chronic KD, self-management program is a preferred method to realize a consistency of awareness, belief and behavior changes.

In this section, we are going to focus on the description of primary prevention of KD.

6.7.1 Selenium Supplementation

Selenium is an essential trace element in human body which plays an important role in body growth and life maintenance. Our previous multicenter intervention trials demonstrated that selenium supplementation has certain preventive effect on the occurrence of acute and sub-acute KD. As to its safe dosage, the recommended daily intake of selenium for a Chinese adult is average 50μg. While in some western countries, according to their diet surveys, actual dietary intake of selenium for one person per day is 31-65μg in the U.K., 70-100μg in the U.S., and 30μg or less in New Zealand due to its low selenium level in soil, respectively.

In practice, oral administration of Sodium Selenite Tablets, originally employed in KD prevention and proved to be a simple and reliable way of selenium supplementation, is troublesome as it needs a specified doctor or a nurse responsible for drug distribution and supervision. Selenium salt, however, very suitable for a wide range of population application, is now being questioned about its safety due to potential carcinogenicity from selenium sulphide impurities. Other options are selenium rich foods and selenium fortified cereal grains. Selenium rich foods include seafood, mushrooms, eggs, etc. But KD areas are almost poor mountainous villages, and local families cannot be affordable for high-price foods. The production of tons of selenium fortified cereal grains can be implemented mainly through spraying aqueous solution of sodium selenate at 0.6 to 1.0 grams per acre over main crops at their heading stage, or by using selenium containing chemical fertilizers. Unfortunately, these two approaches are feasible only in highly mechanized and well developed modern agricultural areas.

6.7.2 Dietary Modifications

6.7.2.1 Soybean and its products supplementation

During 1965-1974, Weihan Yu and colleagues performed a series of community trial in Xinghuo Town of Dedu County and Fanrong Town of Fuyu County, Heilongjian Province, by adding soybean and its products to local residents' food for the prevention of KD (Fig. 6.14).

On a daily basis, either addition of 10% soybean powder to staple corn powder or supply of 275 grams of tofu in subsidiary food for each resident could partially achieve the goal of KD prevention. Since locally grown soybean is easily available in some affected areas, particularly in the northern parts of China, raw soybean or its various dietary products like baby soya-bean milk should be added to local meals in an appropriate proportion.

6.7.2.2 Balanced diet

The dietary structure of people living in KD villages needed to be corrected as early as possible. An investigation showed almost all the children victims in the southwest areas had experienced being fed rice noodle as the only staple food source. In fact, thin pancake of sweet potato and hoecake were also nearly the sole major meals for the people in the central (especially in Shandong Province) and northern affected

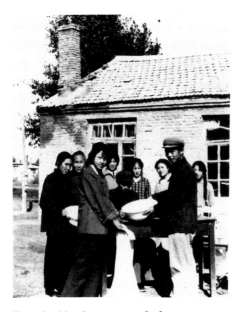

Fig. 6. 14 A group of farmers seen receiving locally grown soybeans as dietary supplement, by which to combat against Keshan disease recommended by Yu's research team, in an undated photo at Fanrong Town of Fuyu County, Heilongjiang Province.

areas, respectively. There were a variety of factors that affected food consumption structure, including short supply of food, income level of families, and food preference.

From the view of disease prevention, the food supply markets and consumption behaviors of residents in KD areas indeed need a nutrition guideline, forming balanced dietary structure through health education campaigns. Under current situation, we would fully realize a reasonable and scientific diet structure by gradually increasing the proportion of soybean products, animal food and vegetables, according to the *Standards for Daily Nutrients Supply* recommended by Chinese Nutrition Society in 1988, as well as referencing to the dietary conditions in unaffected areas.

6. 7. 3　Comprehensive Measures.

The etiology of KD remains unclear, and we should take a consensus strategy of integrated prevention measures based on various etiological views, which has been proved to be effective during a long-term intervention practice in all the affected areas of China. These measures are: (1) to guarantee water supply and quality, to drink clean water; (2) to improve housing conditions, staying away from smoke, moisture, and extreme cold or heat; (3) to keep a good indoor and outdoor sanitation, properly managing human and livestock faeces through fixing corrals and toilets, and better in combination with manure collection activities; (4) to keep stored cereals away from going moldy or getting contaminated; (5) to remove some potential predisposing factors, trying to avoid infection, excessive fatigue, mental stress, and overeating, etc.

6. 8 Surveillance

6. 8. 1 Background

National surveillance of KD began in 1990 at 21 sentinel sites of 10 provinces including Heilongjiang, Jilin, Inner Mongolia, Shaanxi, Yunnan, Shandong, Sichuan, Hebei, Liaoning and Shanxi. During 1995-1999, Henan, Gansu and Hubei provinces joined up to 25 sentinel sites out of 24 counties. On June 18, 1997, Chongqing was turned into a municipality, equivalent to a province, so the total number of the provinces affected by KD became 16. Chongqing, as a new province, was included in the national KD surveillance in 2007. In 2006, the Ministry of Health abolished *KD Surveillance* (*WS/T78-1996*) since KD was well controlled. Instead, a national protocol of KD surveillance was issued. However, the methodology was no substantially different from the original standard. During 1990-2007, the methodology of national KD surveillance was sentinel surveillance, which belongs to non-probability sampling survey. The aim was to find incident cases, to observe the trend of prevalence and the patient's outcome, and to determine risk levels of the people living in the endemic areas where KD was severe historically. Since 2005, the Ministry of Health has expanded the scope of KD surveillance because of a new national public health program. During 1990-2007, the national KD surveillance played an important role in assessing the incidence and prevalence of KD nationwide. In 2008, a national cross-sectional study of KD was conducted using a randomized multistage cluster probability proportional to population size sampling (PPS) methods, to obtain the national average prevalence of KD and its confidence interval estimates. During 2009-2014, the KD surveillance methodology was to continue basically sentinel surveillance, but selected sentinels were based on case-searching instead of the historical data of surveillance. The purpose was to provide sufficient information on the assessment of KD elimination (Fig. 6.15).

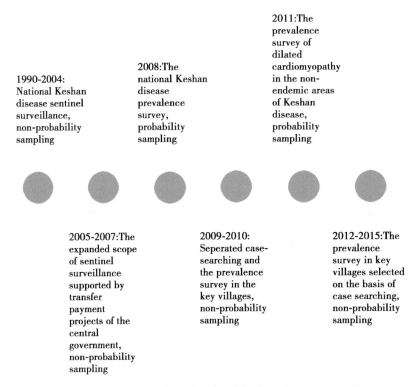

1990-2004:
National Keshan
disease sentinel
surveillance,
non-probability
sampling

2008:The
national Keshan
disease
prevalence
survey,
probability
sampling

2011:The
prevalence
survey of
dilated
cardiomyopathy
in the non-
endemic areas
of Keshan
disease,
probability
sampling

2005-2007:The
expanded scope
of sentinel
surveillance
supported by
transfer
payment
projects of the
central
government,
non-probability
sampling

2009-2010:
Seperated case-
searching and
the prevalence
survey in the
key villages,
non-probability
sampling

2012-2015:The
prevalence
survey in key
villages selected
on the basis of
case searching,
non-probability
sampling

Fig. 6.15 The timeline of national Keshan disease surveillance.

6. 8. 2   What are Involved in the Surveillance Program?

The contents of disease surveillance should include at least three aspects, the incidence and/or the prevalence of the disease, the etiology and/or the risk factors, and the prevention and control interventions and their effectiveness. From 1990 to 2008, KD surveillance was focusing on prevalence and the suspected factor which is mainly the internal and external environmental selenium level of the residents living in the endemic areas of KD, although the etiology of KD is not fully understood. Since selenium deficiency has been widely recognized, selenium level is also considered as a factor that influences the effectiveness of prevention of KD. Residents' income was considered to be an indirect risk. However, during 2009-2012, measurement of selenium levels in the internal and external environment of the residents in the KD endemic areas was not included in the surveillance protocol.

6. 8. 3　How to Monitor Incidence of KD?

In recent years, the surveillance was focused on information collection of the incident cases of KD by using the "cases of young age" concept, which refers to those born after 1980 and are clearly not the cases in which the patients survived from the 1960s through the 1970s. Relatively speaking, the "cases of young age" are "new" cases. The cases of non-transformation originated chronic KD are the same in terms of the epidemiological significance. Both "cases of young age" and the cases of spontaneous chronic KD indirectly indicate the existence of the cause of KD in the endemic areas and the number of these cases further indicates the etiological intensity.

The incident and prevalent status is the key statistical indicator of the epidemic intensity of a disease. As one of the major endemic diseases in China, the indicators of the severity of the KD epidemic should be firstly the scope of the endemic areas, followed by the population at risk, and the incidence, fatality, prevalence and mortality. It should be stressed that not all the classical statistical indicators are applicable to a disease. Incidence is usually applicable to communicable and notifiable diseases. Prevalence, in general, applies to chronic and non-communicable diseases. For years, the key indicator of KD surveillance is to detect the prevalence of KD. The method of KD surveillance is to investigate all the people living in the sentinels (villages) by conducting clinical examinations, and demographic and epidemiological surveys. Clinical examination includes medical examination and electrocardiogram. Cardiac ultrasound and chest X-ray examination are only for those KD-suspected cases that need further to be confirmed.

6. 8. 4　How to Make Accurate Analysis of the Obtained Data and Clearly Demonstrate Results?

Reliable data and appropriate statistical analysis are the keys to provide correct and accurate information on the key indicators such as prevalence and incidence. Another important point is to appropriately present the data and information. These are essential for the policy makers, health care suppliers, media, and residents of the endemic areas of KD to make informed decisions. The core outcomes of the national KD surveillance are prevalence rate, area and age-specific prevalence rates. The detection rates of KD are the "prevalence rates" of the non-probability sampling of the sentinel surveillance. In theory, detection rates cannot be used for making national estimation because its limited representativeness of the residents living in the endemic areas. Because of the probability sampling, the results of the cross-sectional study of KD conducted in 2008 had the estimated national prevalence of KD. It is worth pointing out that quantitative data are often presented in mean and standard deviation, but it is not always the case. For example, the statistical analysis of selenium is exceptional. Being an essential trace element, selenium has toxic effects in case of excess intake. Therefore, the statistical analysis of such quantitative data should (1) display the distribution of data, (2) calculate the proportion of data which are less than the average selenium level of the residents living in the non-endemic areas, and this may be called "Score Lower than the Standard" and (3) calculate the rate or proportion as well as magnitude of the data comparing with the standard.

6. 8. 5   What is the Role of KD Surveillance?

The role of the national KD surveillance is, roughly the same as the surveillance of other diseases, to observe the incidence and prevalence of KD and their trends to provide evidence for policy-maker to design strategy of national KD prevention and control. Prior to 2008, the methods of the national KD surveillance were sentinel surveillance due to limited funding. However, it played an important role in evaluating the incidence and prevalence of KD. Because no case of acute KD and only a few cases of sub-acute KD were found at the sentinel sites during 1990-2007, it was concluded that KD had been well under control. In 2008, a national cross-sectional study of KD with PPS was conducted, which found out the national prevalence and the estimated number of KD. In 2011, a cross-sectional study of dilated cardiomyopathy was conducted among the residents living in non-endemic areas of KD to provide information for the establishment of the baseline or criteria of KD elimination.

6. 8. 6   Quality Control

The quality control of the national KD surveillance requires that, firstly, the scope of endemic areas of KD should be ensured; secondly, the sampling method should be selected in compliance with the surveillance protocol; and thirdly, the data to be collected must be complete for all subjects, especially the clinical examination of the suspected patients, including ECG, echocardiograpphy and chest X-ray film. The response rate of the residents of the sentinels should be no less than 70%. Before the project is started, a training program should be provided to the staff including the clinicians and the field workers of epidemiology. Every day after work, the collected data should be checked in time to find the missing data. The selenium content of the sample in the laboratory detection indicates the experimental methods used in detection and measurement standards of selenium content to reflect the recovery situation. Double entry of data is recommended to avoid data entry errors. Original data should be cleaned to ensure reliable data and results.

6.9　Achievements

6.9.1　Completely Stopped Outbreak of KD in China

Before 1949, the monster KD hit some rural regions in Northern China now and then, and no any effective approaches had been taken to stop it. As reported, this disease ever broke out in sixteen counties of Heilongjiang Province, four counties of Jilin Province, three counties of Liaoning Province, as well as a county of Rehe Province, where the life of affected families was terribly destroyed—a real human tragedy. A survey of Guangrong Town, Keshan County performed in 1935 showed more than 36 people died of this disease within just two months, among a total of 286 local residents. Nearby, according to a villager in Longzhen District, over 700 people in the three villages of interest were killed by an unknown disease like KD in 1927. Afterwards, specific death tolls in 1931, 1935, 1936, and 1941 were documented. Particularly in the winter of 1947, there were more death records than any of the past years, statistically, 1555 being diagnosed with KD from October 1947 through March 1948, of whom 655 were dead out of total population of 4000. On the other hand, in Huanglong County of Shaanxi Province in 1938, there were 40 thousand locals survived this disease out of over 70 thousand people who had moved in for farming reclamation about ten years ago. In Daur Minzhu Town of Buteha Banner, Inner

Mongolia, where KD was prevalent in 1937, 14 out of 24 families in No. 4 village died out, and 6 out of 164 families in No. 6 village became extinct. While in Fushan, a natural village of Arun Banner, more than 300 young women were killed due to an outbreak of KD in the winter of 1944, so earning a nickname 'Single Guy Village'.

During the winter season of 1949-1950, KD swept Northeast and Northwest China again, for example, in Heilongjiang Province alone, 2231 out of 4270 cases newly diagnosed with acute KD were unfortunately dead, with fatility rate as high as 52%. In response to the crisis, the Administration Council of the Central People's Government, now called the State Council of the People's Republic of China, immediately sent emergency medical teams to the affected areas for rescuing KD patients and undertaking epidemiologic investigation, and meanwhile officially requested local governments to conduct related control programs. In 1956, the Ministry of Health instructed to form a National Research Council for KD Control and Prevention which consisted of Beijing Medical College, Harbin Medical University, and Heilongjiang Provincial Institute of Endemic Disease, as well as to establish research bases in some severely affected villages of Heilongjiang. In the same year, a medical team from Harbin Medical University, led by then Associate Professor Weihan Yu, marched into the severe area of KD, and created a combined therapy of rehydration and artificial subhibernation instead of traditional camphor therapy for critical patients with acute KD, significantly raising the cure rate. It was a breakthrough in the history of KD control and prevention. Moreover, in 1958, Yu and coworkers treated chronic and sub-acute patients through expanding home sickbed management mode and a long-term use of digitalis drug together with diet improvement, and achieved a remarkable therapeutic effect.

1950s-1960s of the 20th Century marked the peak of KD outbreak in history, due to the severe damage to people's life in rural areas caused partly by the social movement called People's Communes, and by the 10-year-long Great Cultural Revolution. As a result, the scope of the disease once expanded to southwest area from northern part across middle China, covering 15 provinces including Heilongjiang, Jilin, Liaoning, Inner Mongolia, Gansu, Shaanxi, Shandong, Shanxi, Hebei, Henan, Hubei, Guizhou, Tibet, Sichuan and Yunnan, and more than 30 million people were at risk. Hundreds of thousands of new cases appeared annually, of whom several thousand patients died each year.

Under the close concerns from the Central Government and the direct leadership of the Ministry of Health as well as the North Leading Group of Endemic Disease Control (NLGEDC, formed in 1960s), all participating physicians and health staffs worked together with the involvement of local people. They got a clear picture of the affected scope and prevalence, formulated indicators for the diagnosis and classification, invented mega-dose vitamin C therapy, and summed up emergency guideline " early detection, early diagnosis, early treatment, and on-site rescue" for acute patients. Comprehensive prevention measures included cold-proof, smoke-proof, moisture-proof, drinking water improvement, balanced diet, environment enhancement, and housing condition improvement. In the beginning of the 1970s, most KD areas were turned into status of low incidence.

Since China's open policy in 1978, the introduction of household land contract system in agriculture had sparked an unprecedented fervor of production for allowing farmers to freely plant, and led to steady decrease of KD prevalence in most affected provinces with local economic development. That means, this dreadful disease was dramatically fading away nationwide, and its occurrence has been transformed from widespread outbreaks of acute and sub-acute type to sporadic cases of latent and chronic type. By 1984, KD as an unbridled monster in the past reached its lowest prevalence. Yearly occurrence number of patients with acute and sub-acute KD in the whole country was fewer than 400, of whom fewer than 100 died, indicating the status of the disease was under control.

By analyzing the annual data from the National Unified Surveillance Program of KD since 1990, we found no new acute type case in the past 30 years and no new sub-acute type cases in the latest 10 years across the previously affected areas, suggesting that the prevalence is stably falling. In general, KD in China remains to be sustainably controlled, and in some areas the KD has even been virtually eliminated (Fig. 6.16).

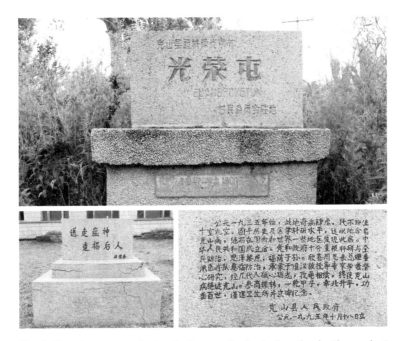

Fig. 6.16 A monument stands for eventual winning the battle against Keshan disease in Keshan County, where the fatal disease was originally discovered.

6.9.2 Built Up a Control System and Working Mechanism

A perfect network for KD control and prevention, including administrative and academic institutions at all levels, had already been formed in all the affected areas during the first 30 years of the P.R. China. From the late 1980s, most professional agencies were merged or cancelled as KD faded away, but a few independent institutions for endemic disease control at the provincial level, as well as some county CDCs (Center for Disease Control) in seriously affected areas was further fortified, with largely updated facilities and instruments and staff training. Regarding the information collection of disease prevalence, we had a report system for acute and sub-acute cases in previous outbreak years, and began to set up an Information Platform for chronic cases based on the Internet since 2015.

In China, a general working mechanism for endemic disease control and prevention is that, government leadership, teamwork of all responsible sectors, and broad involvement of the public as well. It's exceptional for KD control. Achievements largely contribute to the existence of this mechanism.

6. 9. 3 Trained a Large Number of Quality Professionals

In 1964, The North Leading Group of CPC's Central Committee in the Control of Prevention of Endemic Disease made an important decision that KD labs needed to be established, consisting of outstanding faculty members in teaching, medical service and research, in Harbin Medical University, Jilin Medical University and Xi'an College of Medicine, respectively, forming this country's main agencies in KD research.

From 1978 to 2015, Harbin Medical University Institute of KD alone had trained many graduate students, including 67 with master's degree, 36 with PhD degree and 1 postdoctoral scientist. Nationwide, if searching the term "KD" on the website of Chinese National Knowledge Infrastructure (CNKI) to search full-text from "China excellent master degree dissertations database" and "China doctoral dissertations database", there would be 374 with master's degree and 126 with PhD or M.D. degree since 1984. And now, all the graduates wherever at home or abroad are playing their important roles in a variety of job positions. Some of them have become internationally famed experts or senior scientists in cardiovascular field.

6. 9. 4 Made a Remarkable Academic Progress

6. 9. 4. 1 *In-depth Understanding on the Nature of KD*
Over past decades, Chinese researchers have clearly known the scope and prevalence of KD. They were able to understand the etiology, pathogenesis, and epidemic mechanism of the KD through plenty of epidemiological investigations, clinical diagnosis and treatment, pathological morphology, biochemistry, and preventive measures.

In 1973, Weihan Yu gave an updated concept of KD based on available data, concluding that: 1) KD is a chronic cardiomyopathy of unclear origin; 2) the disease demonstrates high-prevalence trend in spatial, temporal and subpopulation distribution of epidemiology; and 3) there are four clinical types of KD, i.e. acute type, sub-acute type, chronic type, and latent type.

6. 9. 4. 2 Effective Ways in Prevention and Clinical Treatment of KD

A safety guideline had been worked out for emergency medical service of KD patients called "three-earliness, and one in situ", meaning early detection, early diagnosis, early treatment, and on-site rescue. Comprehensive prevention measures were summarized as 'Three-proof, and Four-change', namely cold-proof, smoke-proof, moisture-proof, drinking water improvement, balanced diet, environment enhancement, and housing condition improvement. And two primary works: high-dose intravenous vitamin C therapy had an amazing therapeutic effect in rescuing acute patients; and selenium supplementation as demonstrated in many intervention trials was an effective way for the prevention of acute and sub-acute KD.

6. 9. 4. 3 Some New Etiological Theories for KD

Besides active search for better clinical therapy and preventive measures of acute and sub-acute KD, some scientists of our groups also focused on a series of etiological studies. In the 1960s, they successively put forward new views to explain cause of KD, which were generally classified into two categories: chemical factors and biological factors, after ruling out the possibility of Carbonic Oxide Chronic Poisoning speculated by Japanese research teams in the period of Japan invaded Northeast China.

The school of chemical factors argues that the causative substances may exist in soil and water and enter human body through food chain. Shortness or imbalance of certain trace elements, or amino acids, or vitamins would cause an early myocardial injury, while traditional dietary change may trigger the damage. Its main representatives are selenium deficiency theory, and monophagia theory proposed by Weihan Yu. On the other hand, some epidemiologic characteristics of KD, e. g., affected places are usually located in mountainous and hilly areas which are suitable for proliferation of microbes, easy to use biological factors especially enterovirus infection theory and mycotoxin chronic poisoning theory, can explain annual and seasonal high incidence of acute and sub-acute KD. Moreover, some researchers also proposed that multiple factors may be combined by chance under the background of selenium deficiency, which together induces KD.

It is really hard to judge above conflicting theories since every single theory holds its supporting evidences. However, a reliable etiologic clue is that the principal causative agent must be hidden in locally grown cereals, instead of in other media such as water, air, and vegetables simultaneously.

6. 9. 4. 4 Standard System Building

Investigations into KD have been undertaken to provide some guidelines for its diagnosis, treatment and prevention. The criteria originally formulated or revised are listed by publication dates as below:

- *Work Standard for KD Prevention and Control (trial version) [1982-10]*
- *Principles of Management on KD (WS/T 77-1996)*
- *Surveillance of KD (WS/T78-1996)*
- *Diagnostic Standard for KD (GB17021-1997)*
- *Criteria for Evaluating Therapeutic Effect of KD (WS/T 209-2001)*
- *Standard of Pathologic Diagnosis of KD (WS/T 210-2001)*
- *Principles of Management and Criteria of Evaluating Curative Effects of KD (WS/T314-2009)*
- *Control Criteria for KD Areas (GB17019-2010)*
- *Delimitation and Classification of KD Areas (GB17020-2010)*
- *Diagnosis of KD (WS/T201-2011)*

6. 10 Valuable Experiences in Control and Prevention of KD

Since 1949, all levels of government have been highly concerned about harmful magnitude and scope of KD, and speedily dispatched senior medical experts to investigate and control epidemics in seriously affected areas. Owing to great efforts in social mobilization and research, as well as to wide involvement of local residents, we significantly lowered incidence and mortality of the KD via comprehensive measures, and eventually controlled its outbreak despite that the etiology is still unclear. In this chapter, major experiences from national control and prevention of KD are summarized as follows:

6. 10. 1 Broad Political and Social Mobilization

6. 10. 1. 1 Powerful Leadership, Effective Organization and Massive Investment

On December 27, 1949, in the first winter of the People's Republic of China, the former Ministry of Health of Northeast Government dispatched an investigative team to Keshan County, Heilongjiang Province, providing necessary assistance to local residents.

In view of the severity of the disease, local governments put funds to establish specialized agencies and teams for KD control and research, and constantly sent large number of medical workers into the affected villages to provide medical assistance. Moreover, therapy for KD patients was free in some provinces. Sometimes, cotton-padded clothes were also provided for poor relief.

In 1958, the Central Committee of CPC and the State Council jointly decided to put KD into the National Agricultural Development Outline as one of the diseases needing more active prevention and treatment. And in 1960, NLGEDC was formed based on a decision of the Central Committee of CPC, which included KD as one of its key endemic diseases. NLGEDC was renamed as National Leading Group of Endemic Disease Control in 1981, because its function extending to the nationwide. Former chiefs of this organization, included Ulanf, Chen Xilian, and Li Desheng. All of them came from a panel of top power level—the Political Bureau of the CPC Central Committee. An office of NLGEDC, briefly called North Office, had kept playing an important role for 26 years in organizing and coordinating activities of endemic disease control, prevention and research.

Despite being busy, former Premier Zhou Enlai highly concerned about the situation in KD control and research, sent several medical teams into severely affected areas for rescuing patients and investigating the disease cause, spent much time and carefully listened to their work report on KD. Furthermore, former Heilongjiang provincial governor Yilun Wang once instructed Harbin Medical University and Qiqihar Medical College responsible for KD control covering whole province's high-incidence areas, requiring all medical graduates to work for at least two and half months annually in the affected areas.

6. 10. 1. 2　Established a Full-covering Grass Root Control Network Consisting of Visiting Experts, Local Medics and Residents in Affected Areas

In 1953, some medical colleges or universities in Heilongjiang, Jilin, Liaoning, and Shaanxi provinces followed the instructions from the local CPC government, successively sent medical teachers and doctors with rich experiences to the affected areas, performed epidemiological investigations in search for effective therapy, and meanwhile conducted studies on the etiology in combination with the major ongoing work for KD control.

Once again, KD swept the northeast part of China in late 1959.The Ministry of Health of the People's Republic of China immediately dispatched domestic famous experts in epidemiology, parasitology, microbiology, pathology, and clinical medicine, from Chinese Academy of Medical Science, Harbin Medical University, Norman Bethune University of Medical Science, and China Medical University, into the most severely affected regions including Keshan County and Shangzhi County, Heilongjiang Province, and Fusong County and Jingyu County, Jilin Province, to control the epidemic as well as to perform scientific investigation. In these professional teams, there were a number of legendary figures and stories—Professor Weihan Yu has spent 28 Chinese New Year holidays in the severely affected villages to rescue emergent KD patients and to conduct investigations, and was later elected as a member of the Chinese Academy of Engineering; Professor Shichen Wang has discovered an amazing therapeutic effect of intravenous mega dose of vitamin C for acute or sub-acute KD case; Professor Jian'an Tan has created the first geographic atlas of the endemic disease distribution including KD.

During the years of KD outbreak, all involved offices of the leading group for endemic disease control, research institutes, and local medical staff including physicians and public health workers from counties, townships and villages, had worked closely together to form a solid network for controlling KD in the affected areas. In Heilongjiang, for example, provincial governors and secretary of CPC decided in 1953 shortly after being briefed on the disease situation in Keshan County, that in high-risk seasons a command post in every affected county should be established to give immediate instructions in response to reemerging of KD, and meanwhile a patrol member needed to be specified on duty round the clock to send alert once diagnosing a patient with KD, by beating a gong at daytime or lighting up at nighttime, and then doctors in charge would race to save the patient by offering proper clinical treatment.

6. 10. 1. 3 Set up Case Report Rules and Disease Surveillance System

KD isn't classified as one of fulminating infectious diseases, but it always causes local people to be in a blue funk due to its short onset time and high fatality rate. In pandemic period, those medical staffs, who were the first line fighters for KD control in every affected village, were also required to early detect and timely report any new cases of acute or sub-acute KD in attack seasons, besides their usual publicity on comprehensive prevention measures. The case report was required to be submitted in a rapid and step by step way to decision-making agencies. This timely updated information was the most important for proper action, when the KD occurred and emergency treatment was needed.

Since 1990, a national program of KD surveillance has launched, with initial design for detecting new patients in old severely affected areas, and later expanding scope as the increase of funding budget. As a result, the purpose of the surveillance program was not only to find the trend of KD prevalence, but also to search for relatively active areas to ensure the working focus of our efforts.

For years of surveillance, we have obtained a lot of valuable data being used for multiple aspects: first of all, to guide the formulation of national plan for KD control and prevention; secondly, to set our country's technical standards for KD; thirdly, to contribute to timely adjustment of the strategy for KD elimination in China.

6.10.1.4 Adhere to Prevention First Policy

Generally, clinical symptoms persist for victim's lifetime who once suffered from KD, and some severe patients would become disabled, or even dead. So, earlier prevention is always a better choice than medical treatment. In practice, we placed prevention as tenet and top priority both in clinical emergency rescue of critically ill KD patients to avoid death or to turn into chronic type, and in community intervention through selenium supplementation or combined preventive measures to curb potential outbreak of KD. Our next attempts are to find out all important hidden issues by means of long-term surveillance, hopefully to reach a goal of fundamental eradication of KD risk on the Earth.

However, the point needed to be stressed is that in the process of implementing the Prevention First Policy, measures selected for use in eliminating KD should be appropriate to specific circumstances and local conditions of every area.

6.10.2 Strategy Relying on Advanced Science and Technology

How could we have achieved in such a short time the great success in new China from long struggle against KD? The answer is that we insist in exploring practically effective ways for the control and prevention of KD through scientific research.

At the very beginning, most of our physicians could do little for the patients due to limited knowledge of the disease, watching them die in pain. But they eventually found out comprehensive prevention measures mainly containing avoiding coldness, smoke and moisture, drinking water improvement, diet change, environmental enhancement and housing condition improvement. They worked out a safety guideline for emergency medical service of acute and sub-acute KD patients, which is early detection, early diagnosis, early treatment, and on-site rescue. Importantly, the discovery of mega-dose of intravenous vitamin C therapy, use of selenium supplementation, and home sickbed management indeed resulted in remarkable decline of case mortality rate.

There was a milestone event in KD research during 1984-1986, in which 208 participants from 16 institutions took part in an Integrated Scientific Investigation of KD in Chuxiong, Yunnan Province, jointly sponsored by the National Leading Group for Endemic Disease Control and the Ministry of Health. This investigation was carried out in order to search for good indicators in early diagnosis, effective ways of control and prevention, and the pathogenic factors of sub-acute KD. The expert panel led by chief professor Weihan Yu had examined physical, biochemical and pathological morphology aspects of 3648 children who were selected at 10 sites of KD prevalence, obtaining 120,000 analysis data from the total 2397 samples of rock, soil, cereal, blood, hair and urine. The panel won a Second Prize of the Ministry of Health Science and Technology Progress Award in 1990 for their multiple breakthroughs (Fig. 6.17).

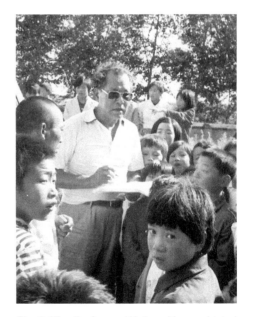

Fig. 6.17   Professor Weihan Yu conducted a survey of school children as part of the Multidisciplinary Scientific Investigation of Keshan disease at Chuxiong 1984-1986.

Also, the Ministry of Science

and Technology, and the relevant departments in some affected provinces have funded numerous research projects on the key problems related to KD control and prevention, during the period of 7th and 8th "5-year state plan". And through these projects, China's works in both control and scientific research of KD have reached international advanced level.

6.10.3 Economic Improvement: a "Once and For All" Control Approach

KD is prone to occur in poor rural areas, where the disease situation always gets worse due to the poverty of local residents, forming a vicious cycle. Based on the previous surveys in some provinces, the decrease of KD prevalence amid outbreak years was largely attributed to great efforts in disease control and prevention, but it was hard to completely control the spread of the epidemic due to epicenter shift. In contrast, since China's open policy was launched in 1978, there have been profound changes in people's working efficacy and lifestyles. With great economic improvement for agricultural population, acute onset of KD has dramatically disappeared nationwide for decades without using any medical intervention in most part of the affected areas.

Specifically, many well-off regions that used to be severely affected areas such as Keshan County, Heilongjiang, and Arongqi, Inner Mongolia, have already changed their risk of KD. However, as typical counterexamples, villages still affected by KD in Qingyang, Gansu Province, are currently still in a low-income state as compared with non-affected rural areas.

Therefore, we strongly recommend that sustainable elimination of KD would work along with poverty-relief programs.

Further Reading

1. The State Technology Supervision Bureau and the Ministry of Health of the People's Republic of China. Criteria for Diagnosis of Keshan Disease (GB 17021-1997). National Standards of the People's Republic of China. Standards Press of China,1998.

2. The Ministry of Health of the People's Republic of China. Diagnosis of Keshan Disease (WS/T

210-2011). Health Standards of the People's Republic of China. Standards Press of China, 2011.

3. The Ministry of Health of the People's Republic of China and the State Management Committee of Standardization. Delimitation and Classification of Keshan Disease Areas (GB 17020-1997). National Standards of the People's Republic of China. Standards Press of China, 1997.

4. The Ministry of Health of the People's Republic of China and the State Management Committee of Standardization. Delimitation and Classification of Keshan Disease Areas (GB 17020-1997). National Standards of the People's Republic of China. Standards Press of China, 1997.

5. The Ministry of Health of the People's Republic of China and the State Management Committee of Standardization. Delimitation and Classification of Keshan Disease Areas (GB 17020-2010). National Standards of the People's Republic of China. Standards Press of China, 2010.

6. The State Technology Supervision Bureau and the Ministry of Health of the People's Republic of China. Control Criteria for Keshan Disease Areas (GB 17019-2010). National Standards of the People's Republic of China. Standards Press of China, 2010.

7. Wang SC. Changing the way of thinking for establishing the therapy of high-dose vitamin C - in memory of the 60 anniversary of the discovery of Keshan disease and the 35 anniversary of the therapy of high-dose vitamin C founded. Bulletin of Endemic Diseases, 1996; (11)2:7-11.

8. Xu GL. Research progress in prevention of Keshan disease by selenium supplementation and the relationship between selenium deficiency and Keshan disease. Bulletin of Endemic Diseases, 1996; (11)2:1-6.

9. Xu GL. The Effectiveness of Sodium Selenite on Prevention of Acute Attacks of Keshan Diseases. Chinese Medical Journal, 1979; 92:471-476.

10. Tan JA, An WY, Li RB. The geo-medical characteristics of Keshan disease. In Keshan Disease Prevention and Treatment in China. Chinese Environmental Sciences Press, 1987.

11. Xu GL, Wang SC, Gu BQ, Yang YX, Song HB, Xue WL, Liang WS, Zhang PY. Further Investigation on the Role of Selenium Deficiency in the Etiology and Pathogenesis of Keshan Disease. Biomedical and Environmental Science, 1979; 10:316-326.

12. Zhu LZ, Xia YM, Yang GQ. Blood GPx Activities of the Residents of KD Endemic and Non-endemic Areas. Acta Nutrimenta Sinica, 1982; 4:229-233.

13. Chen JS. Observations of the Effect of Sodium Selenite in the Prevention of Keshan Diseases. Acta Nutrimenta Sinica, 1982; 4:243-249.

14. Gu BQ. Pathology of Keshan disease. A comprehensive review. Chin Med J (Engl), 1983 Apr; 96(4):251-61.

15. Wang T, Hou J, Li Q, Zhang LJ, Li XZ, Gao L, Pei JR, Deng J, et al. National Keshan Disease Surveillance in 2004. Chinese Journal of Endemiology, 2005; 24(4): 401-403.

16. Wang T, Hou J, Li Q. National Keshan Disease Surveillance in 2005. Chinese Journal of

Endemiology, 2006; 25(4):405-407.

17. Wang T. The Key Issues in Keshan Disease Control. Chinese Journal of Endemiology, 2005; 24 (4): 355-6.

18. Wang T, Hou J, Zhang LJ. National Keshan Disease Surveillance in 2006. Chinese Journal of Endemiology, 2008; 27(3):296-299.

19. Wang T, Hou J, Zhang LJ. National Keshan Disease Surveillance in 2007. Chinese Journal of Endemiology, 2008; 27(4):412-415.

20. Wang T. To Provide Technical Support for Evidence-Based Decision Making in Keshan Disease Prevention and Control. Chinese Journal of Endemiology, 2008; 27(4):355-356.

21. Lavis JN, Røttingen JA, Bosch-Capblanch X, Atun R, El-Jardali F, Gilson L, Lewin S, Oliver S, Ongolo-Zogo P, Haines A. Guidance for evidence-informed policies about health systems: linking guidance development to policy development. PLoS Med., 2012 Mar; 9(3):e1001186. Epub 2012 Mar 13.

22. Elliott P, Wartenberg D. Spatial Epidemiology: Current Approaches and Future Challenges. Environmental Health Perspectives, 2004; 112:998-1006.

23. Zhang GG, Liu Y, Yin XH, Wang T, Ma ZY. Evaluation of the Effectiveness of Chronic KD Patient Self-management. Chinese Journal of Endemiology, 2008; 27:566-568.

24. Rothman, Kenneth J. Modern Epidemiology. Little Brown and Company, 1986.

25. Rothman, Kenneth J. Epidemiology, An Introduction. Oxford University Press, 2002.

26. Elwood, M. Critical Appraisal of Epidemiological Studies and Clinical Trials. Oxford University Press, 2003.

27. Savitz, David A. Interpreting Epidemiologic Evidence: Strategies for Study Design and Analysis. Oxford Univ. Press, 2003.

28. Ahrens W, Pigeot I. editors. Handbook of Epidemiology. Springer, 2005.

29. Rothman Kenneth J, Greenland, Sander, Lash Timothy L. Modern Epidemiology, 3rd. Lippincott Williams & Wilkins, 2008.

30. Centers for Disease Control (CDC). CDC MMWR Guidelines for Evaluating Surveillance Systems. Morb Mortal Wkly Rep., 1988 May 6; 37 Suppl 5:1-18. http:/www.cdc.gov/mmwr/preview/mmwrhtml/00001769.htm accessed as of 2 June 2012.

31. Centers for Disease Control (CDC). Updated guidelines for evaluating public health surveillance systems: recommendations from the guidelines working group. MMWR, 2001; 50 (No. RR-13): page 13-25.

32. Wang T. The Urgency to Harvest the Fruits of Keshan Disease Prevention and Control in Decades. Chinese Journal of Endemiology, 2010; 29(4):357-358.

33. The Ministry of Health of the People's Republic of China. Protocol of National KD Surveillance.

http:/www. moh. gov. cn/publicfiles/business/htmlfiles/mohjbyfkzj/s5874/200908/42374. htm
(accessed on 1 June 2012).

34. Wang T. Translational Epidemiology in Keshan Disease Surveillance. Foreign Medical Sciences: Section of Medgeography, 2012; 33(3):143-147.

35. Ye C, Wang T, Li SE et al. Assessment of Keshan Disease Control in YuanbaoTownship in Shangzhi County in Heilongjiang Province. Chinese Journal of Endemiology, 2015; 34(6):433-436.

36. Wang T. Assessment of Keshan Disease Elimination: Challenges and Opportunities. Chinese Journal of Endemiology, 2015; 34(6);391-392.

37. Zhou HH, Wang T. Progress in the Etiological Studies of Keshan Disease. Chinese Journal of Endemiology, 2015; 34(6):466-468.

38. SUN Dian-jun. Endemiology. Beijing: People's Medical Publishing House, 2011.

39. Yancy CW, Jessup M, Bozkurt B,etc. 2013 ACCF/AHA guideline for the management of heart failure: a report of the American College of Cardiology Foundation/American Heart Association Task Force on practice guidelines. Circulation, 2013 Oct 15;128(16):e240-327.

40. The State Technology Supervision Bureau and the Ministry of Health of the People's Republic of China. Principles of management and criteria of evaluation curative effects of Keshan disease. (WS/T314-2009). National Standards of the People's Republic of China. Standards Press of China, 2009.

图书在版编目（CIP）数据

中国公共卫生：地方病防治实践＝Endemic
Disease in China：英语/孙殿军主编. —北京：人民
卫生出版社，2017

　　ISBN 978-7-117-24713-9

　　Ⅰ.①中…　Ⅱ.①孙…　Ⅲ.①地方病-防治-
中国-英文　Ⅳ.①R599

　　中国版本图书馆 CIP 数据核字（2017）第 148316 号

| 人卫智网 | www.ipmph.com | 医学教育、学术、考试、健康，购书智慧智能综合服务平台 |
| 人卫官网 | www.pmph.com | 人卫官方资讯发布平台 |

中国公共卫生:地方病防治实践(英文)

主　　编:孙殿军
出版发行:人民卫生出版社(中继线 010-59780011)
地　　址:北京市朝阳区潘家园南里 19 号
邮　　编:100021
E - mail: pmph @ pmph. com
购书热线:010-59787592　010-59787584　010-65264830
印　　刷:北京中科印刷有限公司
经　　销:新华书店
开　　本:710×1000　1/16　印张:18
字　　数:313 千字
版　　次:2017 年 10 月第 1 版　2023 年 9 月第 1 版第 2 次印刷
标准书号:ISBN 978-7-117-24713-9/R·24714
打击盗版举报电话:010-59787491　E -mail:WQ @ pmph. com
(凡属印装质量问题请与本社市场营销中心联系退换)